Home Care Nursing

Using an Accreditation Approach

Home Care Nursing

Using an Accreditation Approach

Patsy Anderson, RN, DNS
Associate Professor
School of Nursing
University of Southern Mississippi
Hattiesburg, Mississippi

Deolinda Mignor, RN, DNS
Associate Professor, Ret.
School of Nursing
University of Southern Mississippi
Hattiesburg, Mississippi

THOMSON

DELMAR LEARNING

Australia • Brazil • Canada • Mexico • Singapore • Spain • United Kingdom • United States

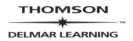

Home Care Nursing: Using an Accreditation Approach
by Patsy Anderson and Deolinda Mignor

Vice President,
Health Care Business Unit:
William Brottmiller

Director of Learning Solutions:
Matthew Kane

Acquisitions Editor:
Tamara Caruso

Senior Product Manager:
Elisabeth F. Williams

Editorial Assistant:
Jennifer Waters

Director of Marketing:
Jennifer McAvey

Marketing Manager:
Michele McTighe

Marketing Coordinator:
Chelsey Iaquinta

Director of Production:
Carolyn Miller

Content Project Manager:
Anne Sherman

Cataloging-in-Publication Data is on file with the Library of Congress
ISBN 1-4018-5233-5

NOTICE TO THE READER

Dedication

This book is dedicated to Gene Mignor and Karen Rich.

Brief Contents

Detailed Contents

Part II: Administrative Operations 131

Foreword

Karen Utterback, RN, MSN, CAN CHCE

Vice President of Clinical Strategy
McKesson Extended Care Solutions Group
Springfield, Missouri

Home Care Nursing—Supporting a New Model of Health Care Delivery

Home health care nursing is in a unique position. We are experts in the management of chronic illness, experienced in the logistics of providing direct client care in the home setting, and challenged by a shrinking pool of available clinicians and the rapidly changing health care environment. An environment where the population is aging, the numbers of chronically ill are rising, and payers are threatening reductions in payment levels while attempting to tie payment to an agency's ability to demonstrate consistent improvement in their clients' outcomes, i.e., Pay for Performance.

How providers choose to leverage their experience and expertise to meet these challenges while continuing to provide outstanding health care will be a deciding factor in their future success or failure. This is not a topic for idle speculation. Home care providers must begin formulating a plan to handle these challenges now. They must consider a paradigm shift away from intermittent care to a care model that sustains optimal levels of wellness, a model where nurses and nursing should be at their best!

In a model focused on sustaining optimal levels of wellness, clients play a greater part in their own disease management, and clinicians monitor clients more closely, enabling them to provide preventive interventions before the client's situation becomes acute enough to require hospitalization or the use of emergent care. Home care providers are depending on technology more than ever to assist them to identify the early signs of decline or exacerbation among their clients. Specifically, they are depending on interactive telehealth technology, electronic health records, and provider and client portals to support their care planning, collaboration, and early intervention, all designed to achieve consistently positive client outcomes.

Changing Demographics Force a Paradigm Shift

The baby boomer generation and the strain it will place on society frequently grab headlines—so frequently that we are inclined to stop paying attention. However, home care providers cannot ignore this unique phenomenon because they are already experiencing the effects. According to recent statistics, baby boomers comprise 28 percent of the total American population—approximately 76 million people (U.S. Census Bureau, Facts & Features). This statistic, coupled with the fact that people now live longer, means that in the near future a far greater proportion of American society will be elderly than at any other time in our history. For the health care industry—and the home care industry in particular—that means a large portion of Americans will need more medical attention.

Chronic illness is known to become much more prevalent as we age. Chronic illness is a disease or condition that lasts for a long period, or is marked by frequent recurrence; for instance, heart failure, chronic obstructive pulmonary disease, diabetes, and asthma lead the list. Today, chronic illness affects 45 percent of the American population. Studies show that caring for people with chronic disease consumes approximately 78 percent of all health care spending in the United States—more than $1 trillion annually (Centers for Disease Control and Prevention, Chronic Disease Overview).

The ballooning population of clients comes at a particularly difficult time for the home care industry. The pool of available clinicians has steadily declined for more than a decade. As a result, home care agencies struggle to find a way to stretch their already over-extended resources to accommodate an increasing number of clients, and it will only become more difficult in the future. Add the continually changing and ever-increasing pressure on reimbursement with demands such as "pay for performance" as well as the growing pressure on agencies to provide high-quality care at lower costs, and the time is ripe for a change.

Disease Management: A New Approach for Home care

Today, home care is focused on transitioning a client from an acute phase of illness to one of self-management, or when a level of independence and safety cannot be achieved, to a higher level of care. Home care services generally are discontinued as the client reaches medical stability, rather than at the point that the client has demonstrated sustainable life style and behavior changes. This model works well if the clients have illnesses that eventually are resolved and if an agency has unlimited human and financial resources in order to manage the cyclical exacerbations of these chronically ill clients. Obviously, these constraints do not reflect today's health care environment. With so many clients, so few clinicians and such a high occurrence of chronic disease that must be steadily monitored rather than resolved, this model is simply inadequate. In a disease management approach, clients at risk are identified early, and care is developed using a collaborative approach involving all members of the health care team and the client. Status of the client is constantly measured. This model has proven to reduce overall expenses, hospitalizations, and the use of emergent care. Medicare is showing signs of recognizing the value of a disease management approach and of home care agencies' integral role in preventing hospitalizations and emergent care use in their chronically ill clients. This is evidenced by the Quality Improvement Organizations (QIO). This is evidenced by the Centers for Medicare and Medicaid Services' (CMS) Home Health Quality Initiative, which includes efforts to encourage telehealth adoption by home health agencies and a focus on reduced re-hospitalization and emergent care rates.

Disease management focuses on long-term health management rather than illness resolution. Disease management programs strive to improve the client's outcomes and quality of life. Not surprisingly, disease management is most effective for chronic diseases, which do not have a cure. The disease management model helps clients alter behaviors, manage their health, and control symptoms by providing client guidance and education. Successfully managing a chronic disease requires:

- an open avenue of communication between the client and caregiver,
- a high degree of client participation in his or her own care, and
- vigilance on the part of the clinician.

A home care delivery model that includes telehealth technology helps home care providers meet these requirements for an effective disease management program. Today's telehealth technology connects the client and the home care provider using an in-home device and an ordinary telephone line. In its most simplistic form, telehealth technology collects client vital sign readings and transmits rudimentary diagnosis information between the client and home care provider. But the technology is capable of much more. Used to its fullest potential, telehealth technology allows the care provider to establish daily, bi-directional communication with the client, transmit clinical content, and monitor every aspect of the client's condition daily. When used in this way, telehealth technology enables more thorough client care than a traditional approach of intermittent in-home visits.

Using Disease Management to Benefit Clients and Providers

By using a disease management program supported by interactive telehealth technology and provider and client portals, home care providers can radically enhance their care delivery system. The benefits of a disease management approach supported by technology are significant to both the client and the care provider.

A successful disease management system helps clients live healthier lives. A program conducted by Sentara Home Care of Virginia found that CHF clients using telehealth with extensive disease management programs experienced an 82 percent reduction in hospitalizations and a 77 percent decrease in ER visits as compared to standard care (Chetney, 2003). By compelling clients to answer detailed questions not only about their vital sign readings, but about their symptoms and knowledge of their diagnosis, providers make clients active participants in their own well-being.

Educating clients about their diagnosis and providing detailed, interactive information helps them to modify behaviors and improve medication compliance. Putting clients in charge of their own care leads to an overall improvement in health, and helps them avoid acute episodes with doctor and hospital visits, which are costly physically, emotionally, and financially. Additionally, going through the motions of answering questions on a daily basis gives clients the comfort of knowing they are being looked after and helps reduce feelings of isolation, which can negatively affect their well-being.

A disease management approach supported by technology helps agencies provide thorough care and conserve personnel and financial resources. It allows one clinician to oversee the health of many more clients than traditional home care visits. Daily updates of client data give the agency far more detailed information about the client's physical well-being as well as his or her emotional health and understanding of self care—two imperative elements to overall well-being that the agency must address for the client to maintain an acceptable level of health. Electronic data collection also helps ensure data integrity and helps the agency maintain regulatory compliance.

Conclusion

Home health care providers are facing a complex set of circumstances—from reduced personnel resources to tighter budgetary concerns. A changing health care delivery model supported by technology is poised to help them meet these challenges. Using technology to deploy a disease management program can help caregivers deliver more proactive client care, education, and support that will empower clients and improve the quality of their lives by allowing clients to control their symptoms for more stabilized maintenance. Home care offers both the expertise and "feet on the street" needed to optimally manage the needs of our aging society. Your interest and commitment to this specialty is essential to the success of our future health care delivery model.

References

Centers for Disease Control and Prevention, Chronic Disease Overview. http://www.cdc.gov/needphp/overview.htm, retrieved Feb 12, 2007.

Chetney, R. (2003). The cardiac connection program. *Home Healthcare Nurse, 21*(10), 680–686.

Health Hero Decision Support Services. Catholic Health care West CHF Program Shows Cost Savings and High Client Satisfaction with Health Buddy and Health Hero iCare Desktop. February 2001. http://www.healthhero.com/papers/studies/CHW_Case_Study.pdf.

Information Technology Association of America (ITAA). E-Health Committee. Chronic Care Improvement: How Medicare Transformation Can Save Lives, Save Money, and Stimulate an Emerging Technology Industry. May 2004. www.itaa.org.U.K. Department of Health. Improving Chronic Disease Management. 2004. http://www.dh.gov.uk/assetRoot/04/07/52/13/04075213.pdf.

U.S. Department of Commerce. Office of Technology Policy (OTP). Innovation, Demand, and Investment in Telehealth. February 2004. http://www.technology.gov/reports/TechPolicy/Telehealth/2004Report.pdf.

U.S. Department of Health and Human Services (HHS). Health Resources and Services Administration and Office for the Advancement of Telehealth. Report to Congress on Telemedicine. 2001. http://telehealth.hrsa.gov/pubs/report2001/main.htm.

U.S. Census Bureau, Facts & Features. http://www.census. gov/popest/national, retrieved Feb 13, 2007.

Preface

"My view, you know, is that the ultimate destination of all nursing is the care of the sick in their own homes. . . . I look to the abolition of all hospitals and workhouse infirmaries. But it is no use to talk about the year 2000."

—Florence Nightingale

Home Care Nursing: Using an Accreditation Approach is designed for anyone who has an interest in home care, from the undergraduate student to the practicing registered nurse. Home care today continues to be a growing and changing market. Many clients who were previously being cared for in the hospital are now cared for at home. The industry continues to grow for many reasons; the aging population, shorter length of hospital stays, and the clinical sophistication of the home care industry itself. Home care agencies are licensed and certified by multiple state, federal, and private organizations. To help provide consistency in the information provided in the text, the Joint Commission (JC), formerly known as the Joint Commission on Accreditation of Health care Organizations (JCAHO), guidelines were selected as the model for organization.

Why we wrote this text

Our goal in writing this text was to offer beginning information on home care in a comprehensive book. As a result we decided to utilize the Joint Commission's outline of standards as the blueprint for this text. This blueprint includes clinical information as well as administrative and leadership topics. Not only is there a need for the undergraduate student to use this textbook but with the growth of the home care industry, there is a need for the practicing home care nurse to have a quick reference. The book can also serve as an orientation tool not only for nurses but other home care staff.

Organization of the text

Home Care Nursing: Using an Accreditation Approach consists of 12 chapters grouped into two parts. These two parts will provide the undergraduate student or practicing home care nurse beginning information about the home care industry. The chapters are arranged as follows:

Chapter 1 presents a history of home care and hospice, its past and present growth, and its relationship to the changing health care environment.

Chapter 2 provides a blueprint for the home care visit, including all related documents for the home care practitioner.

Chapter 3 discusses teaching/learning needs assessment and specifically cultural background, literacy level, and the teaching/learning plan.

Chapter 4 reviews the basic infection control program including tools for infection control, as well as specific clinical implications for home care infections. Several step-by-step procedures are included.

Chapter 5 describes safety in the home and discusses the safety risks involved in the four phases of the home visit. Numerous scenarios illustrate real-life cases and decision-making.

Chapter 6 reviews the client assessment for home infusion, access devices, delivery systems, and client and caregiver information.

Chapter 7 covers agency governance, organizational structure, planning of services, contract design, and financial planning.

Chapter 8 discusses nurse practice acts, client rights, and organizational issues.

Chapter 9 provides an overview of ethics and morality and discusses the nurse's involvement in managing ethical issues.

Chapter 10 presents a comprehensive overview of quality improvement in health care and home care. The chapter includes specific outcomes-based monitoring systems.

Chapter 11 discusses human resource management including methods for recruitment and retention of home care staff.

Chapter 12 discusses the rise of technology in home care including specific technologies and the advantages and disadvantages of each.

Features

Each chapter includes several learning features that provide the readers with a consistent format for the chapters.

- Key terms are bolded and defined within each chapter; all terms are also included in a comprehensive end-of-book glossary.
- Research is addressed through evidence-based practice boxes in select chapters, and also through the literature base underlying each chapter.
- A chapter-closing summary highlights the main points of each chapter. Figures, boxes, and tables illustrate key text discussion points.
- Chapter 5 has safety scenarios to provide additional areas of discussion for the learner.

Acknowledgments

Many people have contributed to the development and publication of this project. We would like to thank our families for their patience and encouragement. We would like to thank our editor Beth Williams and the Thomson Delmar Learning team for having confidence in us through difficult times including Hurricane Katrina. We would like to thank our knowledgeable contributors who were willing to share their experiences with others. We would like to thank the reviewers who made valuable suggestions for the improvement of the textbook.

Contributors

Anna Brock, RN, PhD
Professor
School of Nursing
University of Southern Mississippi
Hattiesburg, Mississippi
Chapter 2: Care and Services

Janie Butts, RN, DSN
Associate Professor
School of Nursing
University of Southern Mississippi
Hattiesburg, Mississippi
Chapter 9: Ethics in Home Care and Hospice

Miriam Cabana, RN, MSN
Coordinator, Learning Resource Lab
School of Nursing
University of Southern Mississippi
Hattiesburg, Mississippi
Chapter 2: Care and Services

Valerie D. George, RN, PhD, CNS
Professor
School of Nursing
College of Education and Human Services
Cleveland State University
Cleveland, Ohio
Chapter 5: Safety and Environment

Kathleen Hoehn, RN, BSN
Health Information Manager
CMC-Home Care
Charlotte, North Carolina
Chapter 4: Infection Control

Jo Johns, RN, OCN, CRNI
Infusion Consultant
Sartin's Vital Care
Gulfport, Mississippi
*Chapter 6: Infusion Therapy: High-Tech
Home Care Concerns and Issues*

Mary Agnes Kendra, APRN, BC, PhD
Associate Professor
College of Nursing
The University of Akron
Akron, Ohio
Chapter 5: Safety and Environment

Andrea McCall, RN, BSN
Director of Quality Management
Post Acute Care Services
CMC-Home Care
Charlotte, North Carolina
Chapter 7: Leadership

Karen Rich, RN, PhD
Assistant Professor
School of Nursing
University of Southern Mississippi
Hattiesburg, Mississippi
*Chapter 9: Ethics in Home Care
and Hospice*

Ralph R. Simone, Jr.
Vice President, Human Resources
Home Health Foundation
Lawrence, Massachusetts
*Chapter 11: Management of Human
Resources*

Jeanie Stoker, RN, MPA, BC
Director
AnMed Health Home Care
Anderson, South Carolina
Chapter 8: Legal Issues

Reviewers

Patricia Chin, BSN, MSN, DNS
Professor
School of Health & Human Services
California State University
Los Angeles, California

Sheila Hartung, RN, PhD
Assistant Professor
Department of Nursing
Bloomsburg University
Bloomsburg, Pennsylvania

Susan Lehmann, RN, MSN
Clinical Assistant Professor
School of Nursing
The University of Iowa
Iowa City, Iowa

About the Authors

Patsy Anderson, RN, DNS, is an Associate Professor of Nursing at the University of Southern Mississippi School of Nursing. Since 1991, she has been a surveyor for the Joint Commission. Patsy has spent the last 23 years involved in the home care industry. She has been the Chief Medical Officer for a home health agency in Louisiana and, for 7 years, was the Director of Home care at Tulane University Medical Center in New Orleans, Louisiana.

Deolinda Mignor, RN, DNS, is a retired Associate Professor from the School of Nursing, University of Southern Mississippi. She has 40 years of nursing experience in a variety of medical-surgical settings, with 10 of those years as a staff nurse for a large home health agency.

Part I

Clinical Operations & Client Care

Chapter 1

Home Care: A Long and Proud History

Patsy Anderson, RN, DNS

Key Terms

Home Care	Joint Commission (JC)	Medicare
Home Health Agency	Medicaid	

Today as health care continues to move away from the inclient hospital setting and into the community and outclient settings, nurses must develop the skills that will be necessary to provide care to clients in these new settings. One of the major areas of client care in this new era of health care is that of home care. Client care outside of the traditional hospital setting is referred to by many names: home care, home health care, hospice, pediatric home health, home infusion, and private duty home care. Even though home care has existed since the time of the caveman, confusion continues to exist as to what home care exactly is and is not. Not only is the general public confused about the definition of home care, but so are many nurse educators and practicing nurses. This book will explore the evolution of home care, identify the component organizations that provide home care, and outline the skills necessary for nurses to provide home care in the 21st century.

For purposes of this book, **home care** will be defined as that component of a continuum of comprehensive health care in which health care services are provided to individuals and families for the purpose of maximizing their level of independence; promoting, maintaining, and restoring health; and facilitating a comfortable death in their places of residence. This definition will allow a discussion of home care that includes home health care, hospice, and pediatric, infusion, and private duty service organizations.

Main Factors Underlying the Growth of Home Care

American society has been aging rather steadily. The rate of aging has varied over the decades, primarily as a result of fluctuations in the rate of decline in the birth rate; fluctuations in the rates and patterns of decline in age-specific death rates; and a shift in the volume and age pattern of immigration. The aging of America will have vast implications in the number of persons requiring special services, participating in various entitlement programs, and requiring formal and informal care. The elderly are not the only clients who receive home care. The home care population includes all demographic types from the very young to the very old.

The United States Census Bureau, in their 2002 report on the 2000 census data, indicated that the growth rate of the total population in the United States more than tripled from the 1990 census report, to 281,421,908. In the 20th century, citizens 65 years and older grew more than tenfold, from 3.1 million in 1990 to 35 million in 2000. Among the elderly population, the growth rate of those 85 years and older was significant, increasing from 122,000 in 1990 to 4.2 million in 2000 (United States Census Bureau, 2002). See Figures 1-1, 1-2, and 1-3.

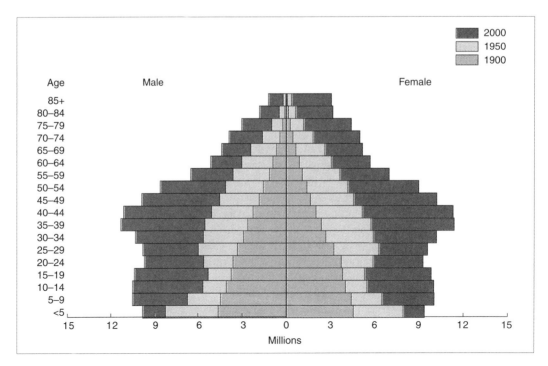

Figure 1-1 Total population by age and sex: 1900, 1950, and 2000. (*Source: U.S. Census Bureau decennial census of population 1900–2000.*)

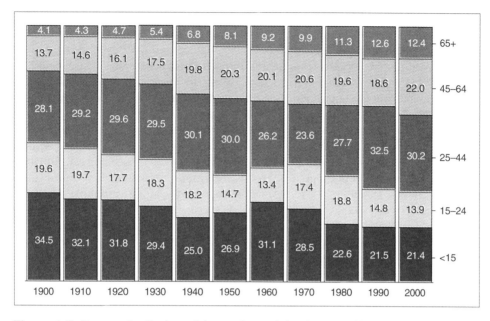

Figure 1-2 Percent distribution of the total population by age: 1900 to 2000. *(Source: U.S. Census Bureau, decennial census of population, 1900–2000.)*

The size of the average household continues to decrease. The average household size declined from 4.6 persons in 1900 to 2.49 persons in 2000. In contrast, the number of single-person households continues to increase. In 1950, 1 of every 10 households was a single-person household; by 2000, 1 of every 4 households was a single-person household. This demographic

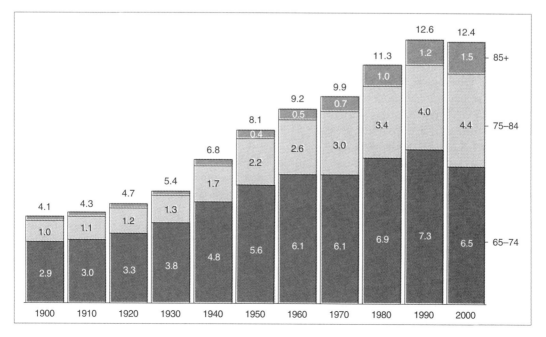

Figure 1-3 Percent of total population age 65 and older: 1900 to 2000. *(Source: U.S. Census Bureau decennial census of population 1900–2000.)*

trend becomes disturbing when there is a need for family support. As the family size continues to shrink, available support for unhealthy family members also continues to shrink. In 2000, approximately 75 percent of all female householders age 65 and over lived alone. As a result, this age group will require support from organizations beyond family that would include home care services (United States Census Bureau, 2002). With the current trend of families requiring both parents to work and the continued rise of the nuclear family, the care of ill family members has begun to depend more on society. With this outside dependence also comes the financial burden of payment for these support services. The median family income in 2004 was $44,389, which was essentially the same as in 2003. At the same time the number of people living in poverty was 37.0 million, up 1.1 million from 2003 (United States Census Bureau, 2005b).

In addition to the current demographic trends, the amount of financial income available to the elderly has begun to fall. In 2001 the median income for all older people was $14,152. Older male income was $19,688 while older female income was $11,313. For 31.8 percent of the elderly, their reported income was less than $10,000, and about 3.4 million elderly persons had income levels below the poverty limit. Another 2.2 million of the elderly were classified as "near-poor." This translates to 16.7 million elderly people who live on annual incomes below $10,000 (Administration on Aging, 2003).

Another health care concern in the United States is the uninsured and underinsured. This category includes people who are referred to as "the working poor," the unemployed, and children without health insurance coverage. In 2001, 41.2 million people, or 14.6 percent of the population, were without health insurance coverage for the entire year. This was an increase of 14.2 percent from 2000, or an increase of 1.4 million people. This number does not include the elderly, who are 98 percent covered by federal programs. The number and percentage of people covered by employment-based health insurance also declined in 2001, from 63.6 percent to 62.6 percent. This change formed the basis for the overall decrease in health insurance coverage in the United States (United States Census Bureau, 2002). The number of the uninsured in this country as of 2004 had increased to 45.8 million (United States Census Bureau, 2005a).

The number and percentage of people covered by government health insurance programs also saw an increase in 2001, from 24.7 percent to 25.3 percent of the total population. This increase was largely due to the number and percentage of people covered by **Medicaid**, the type of health insurance used by the poor. At the same time, the amount of government health insurance coverage did not change for this group from 2000. The proportion of uninsured children remained unchanged in 2001 at 8.5 million, or 11.7 percent of all children in the United States (United States Census Bureau, 2002).

In 2001 health care spending reached $1.4 trillion, which was the fastest growth rate since 1991. Between 1991 and 2000, health care was dominated by managed care organizations rather than traditional insurance plans, and the growth in the quantity and intensity of health care services was slowed as a result. These organizations also restrained health-spending growth by slowing price increases paid to providers and the intensity of services provided. Even with managed care attempting to control health care costs, the growth in utilizations or numbers of individuals accessing the health care systems continues to drive the cost up.

Home Care: A Proud History

For over two centuries, home care in the United States has been considered a natural kind of care, belonging to the family, and associated with the concepts of comfort, compassion, and safety. Families have accepted enormous burdens of responsibility in caring for their sick and disabled loved ones and increasingly have turned to home care providers for help.

The Boston Dispensary in 1796 established the guiding principle for home care: "The sick without being pained by separation from their families, may be attended and relieved at home" (Irwin, 1978, p. 4). They also established the first home care program. During this time in U.S. history, clients were rarely seen in hospitals because they were considered as "pest houses"; that is, once you entered you left in a casket. The clients were taken care of by medical practitioners in the home with the families providing direct client care. The first organized visiting nurse care was provided by the Ladies Benevolent Society of Charleston, South Carolina, founded in 1813. This agency provided skilled nursing care and taught cleanliness and home care techniques to the ill and their families (Hanlon, 1974).

Organized home care began at a time when the most seriously ill were cared for at home; therefore, the home was the workplace for most nurses. The period from 1885 to 1890 was the most dramatic period in the history of American health care. It was a time dominated by infectious diseases and high death rates, while at the same time exciting advances were being made in the medical sciences and public health. Although the origins of the modern hospital also can be traced to this era, sickness was a misfortune experienced by most at home. The arrival of the trained nurse eased the family's burden of caring for the sick at home. They also assisted new mothers by providing necessary prenatal care, helping with home deliveries, and educating the mothers on how to care for their babies. The demand for visiting, public health, and private duty nurses escalated rapidly as their roles gained practical and symbolic appeal.

In 1877, the New York City Mission was the first to send trained nurses into the homes of the sick and the poor. By 1890, 21 visiting nurses associations existed in the United States, each with a staff of about one visiting nurse (Hanlon, 1974). In 1898, graduate nurses were hired by the Los Angeles County Health Department to make visits to the sick poor; the department thus became the first governmental body to provide home care services (Stewart, 1979).

The Henry Street Settlement, founded in 1893 by Lillian Wald and Mary Brewster, was the first organized pubic health agency in New York City. The settlement's services went beyond what is traditionally referred to as public health, for it was Lillian Wald's vision that public health nurses "would be available to those in need in homes, workplaces, in schools . . . and anywhere that people in need lived, worked, played and died" (Hitchcock, Schubert, & Thomas, 2003, p. 30).

Visiting nurses captured the interest of early 20th-century reformers who were concerned that immigration, industrialization, and the infectious diseases of the poor were destroying life in their once-cohesive cities. Many regarded the visiting nurse as the solution to these urban threats. Their brief visits aimed to care for the sick, teach family members how to care for the client, and above all, protect the public from the spread of disease through lessons in physical and moral hygiene. By 1905, 455 visiting nurses were employed by 171 associations (Stewart, 1979).

In 1909, Metropolitan Life Insurance Company, with policyholders in the United States and Canada, began offering home nursing services to its policyholders. It was the first insurance company to offer these services. It also provided the first per-visit payment mechanism for home health services (now referred to as home care services). By 1920, Metropolitan Life had made visiting nurse services available to 90 percent of its 10.5 million policyholders, creating the first nationwide system of insurance payment for home care (Stewart, 1979).

By 1928, home care had become so popular that Metropolitan had affiliated with 953 nursing organizations. Home-based nursing care had reached a turning point and began to decline. Urban death rates were declining dramatically, and chronic, degenerative diseases were replacing infectious diseases as the leading cause of death. Medical, surgical, and obstetrical clients of all economic classes were seeking hospital-based care and private duty nurses followed them into the institutional setting. Although it still existed as an option, home care became increasingly marginal to the hospital-based system that came to dominate American health care. The stock market crash of 1929 precipitated a dramatic decrease in the money available for payment for home care services. As a result, many home care associations, now called agencies, closed their doors in the 1930s (Stewart, 1979).

The growing centrality of the hospital meant that fewer clients were sick at home or required skilled home care by a trained nurse. Many nursing leaders campaigned for the creation of comprehensive, coordinated community-based nursing services; however, the absence of an influential or cohesive constituency prevented them from establishing this type of system.

The rebirth of home care began after World War II, in 1947, with the founding of hospital-based home care at Montefiore Hospital in New York City. Dr. E. M. Bluestone, who found that many indigent people with chronic illnesses were hospitalized for longer periods than necessary, pioneered the "hospital without walls" or "extramural program." Dr. Bluestone envisioned the same hospital staff tending the client in home care with the same clinical record systems and services as those being provided in the hospital. Dr. Martin Cherkasky, the executive director of the program, identified home care services as medical, social, nursing, housekeeping, transportation, medication, and occupational and physical therapy (Ryder, 1967).

Responding to rising hospital costs, an increase in chronic illness, and a rapidly growing older adult population, the home regained its status as a less costly and more appropriate place for care. In 1958, after about ten years of organized home care, the Surgeon General's National Advisory Committee on Chronic Disease and Health of the Aged suggested a national conference be held to discuss the development of home care. The conference, sponsored by the U.S. Public Health Service, was titled "Conference on Organized Home Care" (Public Health Service, 1958). The conference discussed the following concerns:

- Organization of a home care program, including administration, personnel, community resources, and evaluation.
- Standards for development of hospital-based and community-based programs.
- Criteria for the selection of clients.
- Respite services.
- Areas of research and study.

Home care developed in the form of three types of services as a result of the conference: hospital-based home care, community-based home care services, and homemaker services. Hospital-based home care refers to those agencies owned by hospitals. Community-based home care refers to agencies owned by either nonprofit or for-profit companies. Homemaker services are usually provided by community service organizations.

In 1965, Congress passed **Medicare** legislation as part of President Lyndon Johnson's "Great Society" initiative. This legislation provided home care benefits, primarily skilled nursing and therapy of a curative or restorative nature. Certification to participate in the program and to receive federal funding was limited to nonprofit home care agencies and health departments. Based on additional criteria, which required home care agencies to have nursing services and one additional service, of the 1,100 existing agencies providing care in 1963, only 250 would qualify for Medicare participation. Services were expanded in October of 1966 and approximately 1,275 organizations became certified. Therapists, home care aides (formerly called home health aides), social workers, and nutritionists joined the home care team as Medicare provided coverage for these services.

Medicaid, a state medical assistance program for the poor, was also established at the same time as Medicare. Medicaid was established with non-mandatory coverage for some home care services, including nursing and home care aide care and medical supplies and equipment. The Older Americans Act (OAA), a program designed to help maintain and support older persons in their homes and communities to avoid unnecessary and costly institutionalization, also was initiated during this time with some home care funding. Home care had entered its current period of rapid growth (Warhola, 1980).

In 1980 the number of home care agencies certified to participate in the Medicare program climbed to 2,924. One year later, for-profit agencies were admitted into the Medicare Program. Medicare payment for home care increased from $25 million in 1967 to $1.1 billion in 1982 (Parker, 1990).

The National Association of Home Care (NAHC) was founded in 1982 to serve as the American home care community's voice before Congress, regulatory agencies, courts, and the news media. The Association's mission remains to:

- Promote quality care for home care and hospice clients.
- Preserve the rights of caregivers.
- Effectively represent all home care and hospice providers.
- Place home care at the center of health care delivery.

Shortly after opening its doors, the NAHC commissioned the first in-depth market and opinion survey on home care. After discovering that only 18 percent of the American public knew about home care, the association launched a national campaign to heighten public awareness. A 1985 poll indicated that public awareness of home care had climbed to 38 percent (National Association of Home Care, 2001).

According to the National Medical Expenditures Survey (NMES), home care spending totaled $52 billion in 1987, when an estimated 5.9 million individuals, or 2.5 percent of the U.S. population, received formal home care services. Of these recipients, nearly half were older than the age of 65, and the amount of home care they used tended to increase with age. In response to the Medicare denials crisis, in 1987 a coalition of U.S. Congress members, led by Representatives Harley Staggers and Claude Pepper, consumer groups, and the NAHC, filed a lawsuit against the Health Care Financing Administration (HCFA). The successful conclusion of this case in 1989 resulted in a rewrite of the Medicare home care payment policies. These policy clarifications allowed the program for the first time to provide beneficiaries with the level and type of services that Congress originally intended (National Association of Home Care, 2001).

Definitions of Home Care

Definitions of home care are as varied as the number and type of organizations providing the services. A review of these definitions will indicate that they stress either the services provided or fiscal reimbursement. In 1976, the Department of Health, Education and Welfare developed the following definition of home care:

> Home care is that component of a continuum of comprehensive health care whereby health services are provided to individuals and families in their places of residence for the purpose of promoting, maintaining, or restoring health, or of maximizing the level of independence, while minimizing the effects of disability and illness, including terminal illness (Spiegel, 1983, p.17).

Russell, in 1977, defined home care as a general term referring to a combination of health care and social services to individual people and families in their own homes or other community home-like settings. Blum and Minkler (1980) analyzed the types of home care services provided in the home in 1980 and suggested a broad definition of home care instead of the narrowly defined term "home health care." They believed that the policies and procedures for services provided in the home should provide not only for health but also for rehabilitation and independence in one's usual environment. Home health care had been too linked to medical reimbursement patterns, medical definitions, and regulations rather than defining a specific clinical area in which to provide care.

Home care continues to be a diverse and rapidly growing service industry. Today, an estimated 19,690 home care organizations provide health and supportive care services to more than 7.6 million Americans with acute, long-term, or terminal health conditions. This number consists of 7,152 Medicare-certified home care agencies, 2,273 Medicare-certified hospices, and 10,265 home care agencies, home care aide organizations, and hospices that do not participate in Medicare. Annual expenditures for home care are expected to exceed $41.3 billion in 2001 (National Association of Home Care, 2001).

Governmental and Accreditation Organizations

The Center for Medicare and Medicaid Services (CMS) defines a **home health agency** (HHA) (also called home care agencies) as a public agency or private organization, or a subdivision of such an agency or organization that meets the following requirements:

1. It is primarily engaged in providing skilled nursing services and other therapeutic services, such as physical therapy, speech-language pathology services, or occupational therapy.
2. It has policies established by a professional group associated with the agency or organization (including at least one physician and one registered nurse) to govern the services and provides for supervision of such services by a physician or a registered nurse.
3. It maintains clinical records on all clients.
4. It is licensed in accordance with state or local law or is approved by the state or local licensing agency as meeting the licensing standards, where applicable.
5. It meets other conditions found by the Secretary of Health and Human Services to be necessary for health and safety.

In addition to the above requirement, home care agencies must meet the CMS conditions of participation for home care agencies, which will be discussed in Chapter 7. For services under hospital insurance, the term "home care agency" does not include any agency or organization that is primarily for the care and treatment of mental disease (Health Care Finance Administration, 1995).

The **Joint Commission (JC),** formerly known as the Joint Commission on Accreditation of Health care Organization (JCAHO), the national accreditors for health care, defines eligible home care services as those that provide home health, personal care, and/or support services; hospice; medical equipment; and/or pharmaceutical services provided by health care professionals to clients in their place of residence (Joint Commission on Accreditation of Healthcare Organizations, 2002). These health care professionals may consist of nurses, occupational therapists, physical therapists, speech language pathologists, audiologists, medical social workers, dietitians, dentists, physicians, and other licensed health care professionals who visit clients in their homes. Home care services may also include assistance with personal care, activities of daily living, and management of household routine by unlicensed assistive personnel to individuals in their place of residence. Home care services can be provided to individuals in all age groups from infants to geriatrics.

Other types of home care organizations would be those specialty organizations that include private duty services, infusion therapy, and pediatric services. These specialty organizations would provide the same type of home care services as the general home care agency.

Home Care Today

Caring for the acute and chronically ill individual at home has assumed a more significant place in our health care delivery system with expanded services and advanced technology available through home care organizations. More and more people, who at one time would have been confined to a hospital or other institution, are now able to remain at home. In addition to the client choosing to have health care provided in the home, the health care system is now using home care to decrease hospital lengths of stay due to reimbursement based on prospective payment and health care maintenance organizations.

Services range from professional nursing and home care aide care to physical, occupational, respiratory, and speech therapies. Social work and nutritional care, as well as laboratory, dental, optical, pharmacy, podiatry, x-ray, and state-of-the-art medical equipment and supply services, also are provided. Services are paid for directly by the client and his or her family members or through a variety of public and private sources. Public third-party payers include Medicare, Medicaid, the Older American Act, the Veterans Administration, and Social Services block grant programs. Some community organizations provide funding for home care services, as do private third-party payers including commercial health insurance companies, managed care organizations, the Civilian Health and Medical Program for the Uniformed Services (CHAMPUS), and workers' compensation.

In 1992 the NAHC commissioned a poll by Lou Harris and Associates, which found that 89 percent of the American public knew about home care and supported its expansion within federal programs. At this time, spending by Medicare, the largest single payer of home care services, accounted for more than one-third of total home care expenditures. **The Federal Bureau of Labor Statistics reports that new jobs in the home health segment of health care have consistently increased during the years 1996–2005 (United States Bureau of Labor Statistics, 2006).**

While lawmakers engaged in the national debate over health care reform in 1994, the NAHC helped establish home care as a central component to both acute and long-term care in every major plan introduced before Congress. The following year the Center for Medicare and Medicaid Services (CMS) commissioned a project with the Colorado Center for Health Policy and Services Research to assist agencies in implementing outcome-based quality improvement. The key feature of this system would be the Outcome and Assessment Information Set (OASIS). As part of the Omnibus Reconciliation Act of 1997, Congress directed the Department of Health and Human Services to develop a prospective payment system (PPS) proposal. The proposal would overhaul the way home care companies would be reimbursed under Medicare by providing desirable, market-like incentives for the efficient and effective provision of care. This system would be developed with input from CMS, NAHC, and the consumers. See Chapter 7 for a discussion of the Prospective Payment System.

Hospice

Hospice and home care are intertwined; therefore, many home care agencies also have a hospice division. Historically, customs required the family and friends of the terminally ill client to be at the bedside to provide comfort and whatever palliative care was available to ease suffering. Palliative care can be equated with comfort care, and refers to interventions that help to alleviate or lessen the severity of disease or illness without curing or restoring health. Originating in England in the 19th century, early hospices provided palliative care to terminally ill clients in hospitals. Later in the 20th century, services were extended into the home.

The modern hospice concept began in London in 1967. Dame Cicely Saunders founded St. Christopher's Hospice. She believed that the pain of cancer clients could be controlled by administering regularly timed doses of pain medication rather than giving medication only as needed (Beresford, 1993). Hospice care in the United States did not begin until the 1970s. The first hospice in the United States was the Connecticut Hospice, which began service in March of 1974 (Hospice Association of America, 2002).

Hospice care encompasses care that is palliative, supportive, social, emotional, and spiritual to the terminally ill and their families in their home (Hospice Association of America, 2002). The Joint Commission (JC) defines hospice as a program that provides and coordinates an interdisciplinary team to meet the needs of the terminally ill and those with limited life span (Joint Commission on Accreditation of Healthcare Organizations, 2002). The federal government defines a hospice as a public agency, private organization, or a subdivision of either that is primarily engaged in providing care to terminally ill individuals; that meets the conditions of participation for hospices; and that has a valid provider agreement (Centers for Medicare and Medicaid Services, 2005). Choosing hospice care does not mean that the person has chosen to die. At the center of hospice is the belief that every person has the right to die pain free and with dignity, and his or her loved ones will receive the necessary support to allow for that to happen.

The National Hospice and Palliative Care Organization (NHPCO) in 2003 estimated that there were 3,200 operational hospice programs in the United States. Of this number, 2,265 were Medicare certified and 2,368 were accredited by various organizations including JC. For those agencies not certified by Medicare or accredited, the services they provide are regulated by state law.

In 2001, 1,312 hospices were freestanding, 1,024 were affiliated with hospitals, 704 were combined with home care agencies, and the rest were parts of various other health care providers. Hospice admissions in 2001 were approximately 775,000 (National Hospice and Palliative Care Organization, 2003). There were an estimated 579,801 Medicare hospice admissions in 2001 (Hospice Association of America, 2002). In 2001, according to the NHPCO, 2.4 million Americans died, and of those 1 out of 4 received the benefits of hospice care.

Precise information about the total national expenditure for hospice is difficult to determine, but expenditures for Medicare and Medicaid are available (Table 1-1). Using Medicare data, the federal government spent $3.6 billion in hospice care in 2001 (Hospice Association of America, 2002).

TABLE 1-1 Medicare Hospice Outlays, Clients, and Days per Client, Fiscal Year 1989–2001

FISCAL YEAR	OUTLAYS ($MILLIONS)	NUMBER OF CLIENTS	AVERAGE DAYS PER CLIENT	AVERAGE DOLLAR AMT PER CLIENT
1989	205.4	60,802	44.8	$3,020
1990	308.8	76,491	48.4	4,037
1991	445.4	108,413	44.5	4,108
1992	853.6	156,583	56.1	5,452
1993	1,151.9	202,768	57.2	5,681
1994	1,316.7	221,849	58.9	5,935
1995	1,830.5	302,608	58.8	6,049
1996	1,944.0	338,273	54.5	5,747
1997	2,024.5	374,723	50.1	5,402
1998	2,171.0	401,140	47.6	5,412
1999	2,435.1	445,146	44.5	5,471
2000	2,895.5	513,840	47.3	5,635
2001	3,610.7	579,801	49.9	6,228

Source: CMS, Office of the Actuary, Center for Health Plans and Providers (September 2002).

Medicare and Hospice

Congress, in November of 1983, legislated a Medicare hospice benefit for reimbursement to Medicare-certified hospice agencies (Health Care Finance Administration, 1984). The legislation called for termination of the program in September of 1986. In April 1986, public law 99-272 was enacted and made the hospice benefit a permanent Medicare benefit. The law held that terminally ill Medicare beneficiaries with a life expectancy of 6 months of less would be eligible for hospice services. With enactment of the Balanced Budget Act of 1997, the Medicare hospice benefit was changed to more specific time periods.

The periods were:

- An initial 90-day period.
- An additional 90-day period.
- An unlimited number of additional 60-day benefit periods as long as the client continues to meet program eligibility requirements (Hospice Association of America, 2002).

Hospice health care professionals and services may consist of:

- Nurses
- Physicians
- Clergy

- Therapy services
- Volunteer services
- Home care aides and homemaker services
- Counseling services
- Drugs for pain control and symptom control
- Medical equipment and supplies

Hospice services can be provided not only in the home but also in an inclient facility. When admitted to an inclient facility, a hospice organization can provide short-term inclient care. This care may be provided in a designated hospice inclient unit, or a participating skilled nursing facility or nursing home facility that meets the special hospice standards regarding client care and staffing areas. A hospice may not arrange to provide inclient services to a Medicare beneficiary in a Veterans Administration or military hospital because Medicare cannot pay for services for which another government agency has paid or is obligated to pay. Services provided in an inclient setting must conform to the written plan of care (Centers for Medicare and Medicaid Services, 2005). When the client's condition worsens, he or she can be maintained at home; continuous home care can be provided during a period of crisis. A period of crisis is identified as a period in which a client requires continuous care which is primarily nursing care to achieve palliation or management of acute medical symptoms. If a client's caregiver has been providing a skilled level of care for the client and the caregiver is unwilling or unable to continue providing care, this may precipitate a period of crisis because the skills of a nurse may be needed to replace the services that had been provided by the caregiver.

In hospice, the family members provide a large amount of client care and at some period that family may need a break from client care. In these situations hospice care can provide for respite care. Respite care is short-term inclient care provided to the individual only when necessary to relieve the family members or other persons caring for the individual at home. Respite care may be funded only on an occasional basis.

The Medicare hospice benefit requires that the hospice organization provide bereavement counseling for a period of at least one year after the client's death. Bereavement counseling consists of counseling services provided to the individual's family after the death of the individual (Centers for Medicare and Medicaid Services, 2005).

Hospice organizations are required to provide core services to qualify for federal and state payment. These core services would include nursing, medical social services, and counseling (Centers for Medicare and Medicaid Services, 2005).

The Newest Home Care Services

With the changes in medical care and reimbursement, more types of home care are being provided. Some of the newest home care organizations are pediatric services, infusion therapy, durable medical equipment, and private duty and personal care. Pediatric home care services are programs designed exclusively for infants, children, and adolescents (Box 1-1). These programs may provide supplies and equipment either directly or through contracts with other organizations.

Over the past 20 years, home care infusion services have continued to expand. In the 1980s home infusion consisted of IV hydration and total parenteral nutrition. It now includes many other types of therapies once provided only in the hospital setting (Box 1-2).

BOX 1-1 PEDIATRIC HOME CARE SERVICES

- Nursing
- Home infusion
  - IV antibiotics
  - TPN therapies
  - Chemotherapy
  - Hydration
  - Growth hormone
  - Factor VII
  - Pain management
  - All other infusion types
- Medical Equipment
  - Phototherapy blankets
  - Apnea monitors
  - Enteral Nutrition
  - Oxygen
  - Ventilators
  - Suction equipment
  - All other durable medical equipment
- Ancillary personnel
  - Physical therapists
  - Occupational therapists
  - Speech therapists
  - Respiratory therapists
  - Social worker
- Managed care programs
  - Hospice
  - AIDS
  - Cystic Fibrosis
  - Other types of specialty programs

With more organizations providing health care services at home, a recent entry into the home care market has been that of the durable medical equipment (DME) industry. This type of organization is the largest supplier of respiratory care equipment in the home (Box 1-3).

BOX 1-2 HOME CARE INFUSION SERVICES

- Nursing
  - Administration of drug therapies
  - Health assessment
  - Adverse drug reactions and side effects management
  - Client education
- Pharmacists
  - Medication dispensing and preparation
  - Clinical drug monitoring
  - Client care planning
- Therapy types
  - IV antibiotics
  - Total parenteral nutrition (TPN) therapies
  - Chemotherapy
  - Hydration
  - Growth Hormone
  - Factor VIII
  - Pain management
  - AIDS related therapies
  - Inotropic Therapy
  - Tocolytic therapy
  - All other infusion types
- Infusion pumps and tubing
- Nutritional support
- Laboratory analysis
- Delivery of medication, supplies, and equipment

BOX 1-3 MEDICAL EQUIPMENT SERVICES

- Respiratory services
  - Oxygen concentrators
  - Liquid oxygen
  - Portable oxygen
  - CPAP and BiPAP machines
  - Compression nebulizers
  - Home ventilators
  - Noninvasive ventilator support (NVS)
- Equipment
  - Hospital beds and accessories

- Bathroom aides
- Wheelchairs, canes, and walkers
- Client lifts
- Home phototherapy and apnea monitors
- Enteral nutrition
- Ongoing maintenance of equipment
- All other types of medical equipment

One of the newest services provided by the DME organizations is continuous positive airway pressure (CPAP). CPAP devices maintain open airways in clients suffering from obstructive sleep apnea by providing airflow at prescribed pressures during sleep. The home ventilator is now becoming a much smaller and more easily managed piece of respiratory equipment. The types of ventilators used in the hospital setting are much larger than those used in home care today. These state-of-the-art ventilators combined with clinical experience, education, and training of the family can provide a stable environment for the ventilator-dependent client. This equipment is also portable enough to allow the ventilator-dependent client to leave the home. Another new service being provided DME organizations is customized mobility systems, seating and positions systems, adaptive equipment, and orthotic and prosthetic appliances.

One of the oldest types of home care and nursing care is that of private duty and personal care. Nursing before the advent of the institutional setting was all private duty nursing. The private duty nurse was paid by the family. Today private duty and personal care is making a comeback, and is now paid for by insurance companies. Today an estimated 13 million Americans of all ages need assistance to carry out daily activities. With the continued graying of America, this number will continue to rise. The private duty organization will provide nursing care services and personal care on an hourly basis. These services are not required to be skilled in nature (Box 1-4).

BOX 1-4 PRIVATE DUTY AND PERSONAL CARE

- Nursing
  - All skilled services
  - Medication administration and monitoring
  - Medical observation
  - Rehabilitation services
  - Telephone reassurance
  - Alzheimer's and dementia care

- Personal care and support
  - Bathing and dressing
  - Ambulation
  - Respite care
  - Incontinence care
  - Live-in services
  - Grooming and hygiene
  - Companionship
  - Daily activities assistance

Summary

Home care will continue to grow and change as it has over the past two centuries. As the health care system continues to change and mature, so will the home care industry. Today home care is providing client services that could not have been imagined even in the 1970s. It will be necessary for nursing to stay in the forefront of the home care industry, because the largest number of home care services are provided and supervised by the nurse.

References

Administration on Aging. (2003). *Income and poverty among the elderly.* April 9, 2003.
   http://www.aoa.gov

Beresford, L. (1993). *The hospice handbook: A complete guide.* Boston: Little and Brown.

Blum, S. R., & Minkler, M. (1980). Toward a continuum of caring alternatives: Community based care for the elderly. *Journal of Social Issues, 36*(2), 133-152.

Centers for Medicare and Medicaid Services. (2005). *Hospice manual* (Publication No. 11). January 23, 2003.
   http://www.cms.hhs.gov/manuals

Hanlon, J. J. (1974). *Public health administration and practice* (6th ed.). St. Louis: C.V. Mosby.

Health Care Financing Administration. (1984). Medicare program: Hospice care. *Federal Register 48*(560008-36). Washington, DC: Government Printing Office.

Health Care Financing Administration. (1995). *Home care insurance manual* (Publication No. 11). Washington, DC: Department of Health and Human Services.

Hitchcock, J. E., Schubert, P. E., & Thomas, S. A. (2003). *Community health nursing: Caring in action* (2nd ed.). Clifton Park, NY: Thomson Delmar Learning.

Hospice Association of America. (2002). *Hospice facts & statistics.* February 1, 2003.
   http://www.nahc.org

Irwin, T. (1978). *Home care: When a client leaves the hospital.* New York: Public Affairs Committee.

Joint Commission on the Accreditation of Healthcare Organizations. (2002). *2003 Comprehensive accreditation manual for home care.* Oakbrook Terrace, IL: Joint Commission Resources, Inc.

National Association of Home care (NAHC). (2001). *Basic statistics about home care.* February 1, 2003.
   http://www.nahc.org

National Hospice and Palliative Care Organization. (2003). *NHPCO facts and figures.* Arlington, VA: National Hospice and Palliative Care Organization.

Parker, M. (1990). How to succeed in the home care business in the 1990's. *Caring, 9*, 8-14.

Public Health Service. (1958). Chronic disease program. *Report of the Roanoke Conference on Organized Home care.* Washington, DC: Government Printing Office.

Russell, D. L. (1977). Home care—another way to reduce costs? *Pennsylvania Medicine, 80*, 9–22.

Ryder, C. F. (1967). *Changing patterns in home care* (Publication No. 1657). Washington, DC: Public Health Services.

Spiegel, A. D. (1983). *Home healthcare*. Owings Mill, MD: National Health Publishing.

Stewart, J. E. (1979). *Home care*. St. Louis: C.V. Mosby.

United States Census Bureau. (2000). *Demographic trends in the 20th century.* September 30, 2002.
http://www.census.gov

United States Census Bureau. (2002). *Health insurance coverage: 2001.* September 30, 2002.
http://www.census.gov

United States Census Bureau. (2005a). *Census Bureau uninsured number indicates fourth increase in a row*. August 30, 2005.
http://www.census.gov

United States Census Bureau. (2005b). *Number in poverty and poverty rate: 1959–2004.* August 30, 2005.
http://www.census.gov

United States Department of Labor, Bureau of Labor Statistics. (2006). *Employment, hours, and earnings from the current employment statistics survey (national): Home health-care services*. retrieved 10/2/06 from
http://data.bls.gov/PDQ/servlet/SurveyOutputServlet:jsessionid=f030f6682e85$2D$3F$1

Warhola, G. (1980). *Planning for home care services: A resource handbook* (Publication No. HRA 80-12017). Washington, DC: Department of Health and Human Services.

Chapter 2
Care and Services

Anna Brock, RN, PhD
Miriam Cabana, RN, MSN

Key Terms

Certification	Outcomes and Assessment Information Set (OASIS)	Referral
Home Care		Skilled Care
	Plan of Care	

Home care can be defined as that component of a continuum of comprehensive health care in which health care services are provided to individuals and families for the purpose of maximizing their level of independence; promoting, maintaining, and restoring health; and facilitating a comfortable death in their places of residence. Refer to Chapter 1 for an in-depth discussion of home care definitions. The key to achieving this goal is to coordinate all services available within the home care agency (also called home health agency) and community.

This chapter will focus on care and services offered to clients in the home and community setting. Topics to be covered include the role of home care providers, the coordination of services, the home care nurse visit, challenges in home care nursing care, and discharge planning.

Disciplines and Roles

Quality home care delivery involves a partnership among many disciplines. The needs of the client and family must be determined through the collaborative and cooperative efforts of these professional and technical health care providers. The various professional providers see clients separately and get together to coordinate the plan of care while administrative and clerical staff provide support from the office. All health care providers work to assist the client to regain his or her state of wellness and self-care, promoting independence to assist the client to remain in the home for as long as possible. The most common disciplines found in home care and their roles will be discussed.

Physicians

Physicians must be a licensed doctor of medicine, podiatry, or osteopathy in order to refer clients to home care and to write orders for home care (National Association for Home Care, 1996; Community Health Accreditation Program, 2002). All skilled and unskilled care and services provided to home care clients must be certified by a physician's order. The physician's signature on the plan of care certifies that the client does have a medical problem that requires the skills and services ordered. Physicians provide orders for care as required by assessment reports from home care nurses or following physician assessments during office visits.

Registered Nurses

Home care agencies employ registered nurses (RNs) prepared at the diploma, associate, baccalaureate, and master's levels. The American Nursing Association (ANA) developed standards of home care nursing practice in the 1980s to ensure the delivery of quality nursing care (refer to Chapter 8 for a discussion of standards of practice). Diploma, associate, and baccalaureate-prepared nurses usually function in the role of staff nurse, while administrators and clinical specialists are prepared at the master's level. Advanced practice nurses (master's prepared) who function as clinical specialists in their respective areas of interest (for example, oncology, psychiatry) may serve as resources and consultants for other nurses, manage a specialty within an agency, serve as case managers for clients with complex needs, and provide expert skills for clients who have particular needs for their services.

Home care agencies also employ or contract with registered nurses who are certified in specialty areas. The most common are the enterostomal therapists (ETs), who specialize in skin care, wound assessment and treatment, and ostomy teaching and care; cardiovascular nurses; and infusion therapists who are certified in peripherally inserted central catheters (PICCs), ports, and Broviac/Hickman and Groshong catheters. The availability of these nurses in the home can help reduce complications, mortality, re-hospitalizations, and most importantly, allow clients to remain in their own environment (Humphrey, 2002).

Home care nursing has a scope of practice that is different from any other nursing specialty. There is a high level of autonomy in home care nursing. Home care nurses must demonstrate a high level of competency in assessment; complex technical clinical skills; problem-solving, critical thinking, and clinical decision-making skills; and strong organizational skills. The home care nurse must be able to effectively teach the client and caregiver to promote wellness and self-care, recognize and assist with medication management, and provide culturally congruent care. Further, competence, experience, and knowledge about regulatory mechanisms; how to interpret skilled care needs; and how to provide the objective data to account for the services to third-party payers are essential components of the home care nurse's repertoire.

Registered nurses function as primary care nurses, case managers, and team leaders. When occupational therapy and social work services are the only skilled disciplines required for a client, the RN must be assigned as the primary nurse or case manager. Physical therapy and speech and language therapy, on the other hand, can "stand alone." That is, the registered physical therapist (RPT) can admit and case-manage a client when there are no nursing skills required (U.S. Department of Health and Human Services, 2000).

Registered nurses are responsible for the comprehensive admission assessment, planning and implementing an initial educational plan for the client and caregiver, and developing and documenting a care plan with the client and caregiver. Most home care agencies have abolished the "admissions nurse" and have opted to assign admissions to primary nurses as the referrals arrive or by geographic location of the client to be admitted. All nurses must be proficient in the admission process. The primary nurse is responsible for the treatment plan implementation, ongoing assessments, assessments when any significant change occurs in the client's condition, and recertification assessments.

Typically the RN in home care is a case manager, client advocate, change agent, and care coordinator. The RN communicates with the client/caregiver and any other entity that affects the client's care, including the client's family, other nurses involved in care, the aide, the physician, therapists, the pharmacist, third-party payers, and medical equipment and supply companies. Nursing care delivery models in which the case manager or utilization manager is not used to coordinate the client's care require the primary nurse to report outcomes, request visits, and otherwise collaborate with third-party payer case managers.

Licensed Practical or Vocational Nurses

Licensed practical or vocational nurses (LPN/LVNs) may work in home care within the framework of state nurse practice acts and licensing boards. These nurses may perform technical skills (such as assessment, wound care) and reinforce teaching initiated by the RN. Many home care agencies employ these nurses as office nurses who take physician phone orders and communicate the orders to the RN responsible for each client. LPNs/LVNs cannot serve as a client's primary nurse or case manager. Each agency provides these practitioners with supervision by an RN (Community Health Accreditation Program, 2002).

Therapists

Home care agencies employ registered therapists to provide therapy in the home of clients who are unable to travel to outpatient clinic settings. A physician's order and an appropriate diagnosis that indicates the need for therapy is required. Therapists are responsible for developing a plan of care with outcome goals for the physician and third-party payers (Medicare, insurance companies) for reimbursement. Home therapy has the primary goal of assisting the client to become as independent as possible within the limitations of the disease state, modify the environment to ensure safety and promote independence, and increase functional abilities.

Physical Therapists   Registered physical therapists (RPTs), who are educated at least at the baccalaureate level and must hold state licensure, assist clients with ambulation and transferring, and teach muscle-strengthening exercises and balance and transfer techniques. RPTs assess the client's environment for modifications that can facilitate or maintain safety and promote increased functional abilities. The assessment is then communicated to the care manager and/or the physician. A physician's order is required for the equipment and therapy plans.

RPTs estimate the time period therapy is required, any equipment needed to attain the desired outcome, and the prognosis for obtaining the desired outcome. The RPT performs the initial comprehensive assessment for clients who require only therapy. RPTs may work alone with the client and/or caregiver or with the RN and home care aide to provide safety and progress toward therapy goals (Anemaet et al., 2001).

Physical therapy assistants (PTAs) are frequently employed by home care agencies and are supervised by the RPT. The PTA must have either a two-year degree from an approved program or two years' experience as a PTA and have successfully passed a proficiency exam. The PTA is provided with specific instructions for treatment and follows the treatment plan developed by the RPT. The RPT must be available by phone when the PTA is in the client's home.

Occupational Therapists   Occupational therapists (OTs) are baccalaureate-prepared and board-certified therapists who work with home care clients to improve their upper body strength and to teach them to use assistive devices to enhance independence. They help clients find alternate ways of managing activities of daily living (ADLs) and help solve problems that increase risk for injury or interfere with the goal of independence. There must be a physician's order for the OT to visit the client and for any devices the therapist deems necessary for the client. Occupational therapists are not a qualifying service for Medicare clients but can only begin if nursing or physical therapy is also seeing the client.

Speech/Language Therapists   Speech/language therapists (SLTs) are master's-level prepared and are state-licensed therapists who work with clients who have swallowing difficulties, cognitive speech problems, functional speech impairments, and voice and language disorders. Some of the most common medical diagnoses that are associated with the need for ST services are stroke, head trauma, dysphagia, throat cancer, and Parkinson's disease. A physician's order is required to initiate these services. Speech and language is a qualifying service; therefore, nursing and physical therapy services are not required for initiation of speech and language services (Brown, Hasselkus, and Tenenholtz, 2002; Centers for Medicare and Medicaid Services, 2005).

Social Workers

Social workers (MSWs) must be prepared with a master's degree in social work to work in the home care setting. Each agency determines the amount of experience required for employment. The MSW must have a physician's order to enter the client's home; however, social worker visits are not a qualifying service for Medicare clients but can only begin if nursing or physical therapy is seeing the client. Social workers assist home care clients and caregivers to locate community resources the client needs when admitted to home care or those the client needs upon discharge from home health. They also assist clients in applying for services or link them to services. Home-delivered meals, homemaker services, support groups, and short-term counseling are but a few of the services social workers coordinate. Long-term care counseling and placement and caregiver issues are also addressed by the MSW. The MSW usually visits the client once or twice during the 60-day certification period. Additional visits for follow-up must be requested from the physician and an order received and documented.

Home Care Aides

Home care aides, also called home health aides (HHAs), are highly visible and vital members of the home care team. Aides see the client more frequently than any other home care provider and are often the first to identify a client problem, which they communicate to the

RN. Home care agencies approved to receive Medicare reimbursement hire only those aides trained and state certified as home care aides. The home care aide either completes a certification program or successfully completes a skills competency evaluation (Bull and Halligan, 2002). Home care agencies accredited by the Joint Commission (JC) are held to the same requirements for home care aide preparation as the Medicare Conditions of Participation.

The home care aides are responsible for providing temporary personal hygiene, assessing vital signs, providing a safe and clean environment with light housekeeping (particularly in the client's bedroom), reinforcing self-care teaching, assisting with RPT/OT exercise plans, and occasionally preparing light meals. The home care aides can remind clients to take their medications, but they cannot administer the medications. The RN or RPT must request an order for the aide from the physician and justify the need for home care aide services. Their visits must be intermittent (in the home fewer than eight hours/day). RNs or RPTs directly supervise the home care aides. The home care nurse or RPT must meet the aide in the client's home for the initial home care aide visit; this constitutes the first supervised aide visit. The aide's plan of care is developed with the client, caregiver, nurse/therapist, and aide. The plan is specific about the types of care the aide is to provide, safety measures, observations to report to the nurse/therapist, the frequency of visits, as well as the days and times those visits are to occur, and any preferences the client may express.

The RN or RPT must supervise the home care aide every two weeks. Two weeks following the initial aide supervised visit, the RN or RPT makes an unsupervised aide visit. Thereafter, supervised visits are scheduled at least every 60 days and following any inclient stays, and unsupervised visits are scheduled every two weeks until the client is discharged. The unsupervised aide visit is made in the absence of the aide; and the client and caregiver are asked to evaluate the care they receive from the aide. Some agencies allow a nonchargeable visit for the nurse/therapist to evaluate the aide when a skilled visit is not scheduled during the evaluation period.

Durable Medical Equipment Companies

Durable medical equipment (DME) companies are privately owned or corporate medical equipment and supply companies that provide home care equipment, such as feeding pumps and tubing, feeding formula, hospital beds, pressure-reducing mattresses, oxygen, and even ventilators. When this type of equipment is needed, a physician's order is required in order to bill third-party payers. The DME company usually sends a representative to the home to teach the client, caregiver, and nurse how to operate the equipment. Other supplies required to provide care to the client are ordered by the home care office and are distributed to the client during the nurse, aide, or therapy visits. A physician's order is required for supplies that may include diapers, catheters, saline, sterile gauze, and tape. The client's payer will individually determine reimbursement for medical supplies.

Plan of Care and Physician's Orders

Home care and services are initiated only by a physician's order. Home care services can only be provided under the supervision of a licensed doctor of medicine, podiatry, or osteopathy and if the client meets the criteria for home care required by their payer source. Most payer sources generally follow the Medicare guidelines; however, for self-paying clients, all that is needed is the physician's order. The physician's order for a client assessment or evaluation for the need of skilled home care (nursing or therapy) is commonly called a **referral.** The referral may be called to the home care office from the physician's office or clinic, or a nurse or social worker responsible for discharge planning from an acute care, skilled care, or rehabilitation facility may notify the agency of the referral. The verbal phone order is followed by a written order that is sent by fax to the home care office and placed on the client's chart.

The referral must be received by a nurse (RN or LPN/LVN). Some agencies assign one office nurse as an intake nurse, a case manager, team leader, or coordinator to accept and to communicate the referral to the appropriate person (Humphrey, 2002). There is usually an agency-specific intake or referral form used to record the data. The information may include minimal demographic data (name, age, birthday, gender, address, phone number, Medicare or Medicaid number, and Social Security number); an emergency contact person; diagnosis or diagnoses; dates of acute care, skilled care, or rehabilitation stays or onset of illness; new or changed medications; and any specific assessment or procedure orders, such as wound care protocol. If adequate information is provided, the payer source can be verified prior to the initial visit. If there is no known payer source, the referral needs to be directed to the office manager or administrator. Referrals for clients who are to receive infusion therapy or high-tech care require more detailed information. The referral may include a desired frequency of visits by the nurse or therapist; or more commonly, the referral may be general, such as "evaluate for home health."

A copy of the referral is given either to the person who coordinates or assigns admission assessments (depending on the delivery model) or directly to the nurse or therapist who will conduct the assessment the following day. In accordance with most agency policies, the initial comprehensive evaluation is completed within 24 to 48 hours after the referral is received. This timeframe can be superseded by the need for complex care on the same day the client is discharged from a facility (such as the need for a ventilator) or if a homebound client has an acute onset of a health problem.

The nurse or therapist assigned to conduct the initial visit is responsible for calling the client/caregiver to obtain directions to the home, to arrange a time for the visit, to explain the usual length of the initial visit (approximately 1½ to 2 hours), and to inform the client/caregiver that insurance cards, medications, and discharge summaries will need to be available for the nurse's or therapist's review. The nurse or therapist will visit the client to assess the need for **skilled care.** Skilled care is defined as care that only a registered nurse or registered physical therapist can provide. The nurse or therapist must be knowledgeable about the payer source requirements for the client to receive home care and services (for example, Medicare requires the client to be homebound, require skilled care, and care must be intermittent).

The nurse or physical therapist (for therapy-only orders) performs a comprehensive assessment of the client and the environment for the start of care. Each Medicare-certified home care agency has been mandated to integrate the **Outcomes and Assessment Information Set (OASIS)** data set into the client's initial assessments (Krulish, 2000). OASIS will be fully discussed later in this chapter. The comprehensive assessment for the start of care is conducted using the agency admission form that includes the OASIS items that will measure three dimensions from the data collected: the clinical status, functional status, and service utilization. This information is then used to determine the dollar amount of reimbursement the agency will receive (for Medicare recipients) as well as the disciplines that need to be included in the client's care. The completed assessment form is forwarded to a nurse who is responsible for scrutinizing each portion of the comprehensive assessment form for accuracy;

completeness; appropriate, correct, and specific primary and secondary diagnostic ICD-9 codes; disciplines and frequencies; and to ensure compliance with the prospective payment system (PPS) for Medicare recipients to make certain that the maximum allowable reimbursement is received. The physician's orders, comprehensive assessment, available agency reimbursement, treatment needed, and disciplines necessary to deliver the treatment are combined into a client plan collectively referred to as the **plan of care.**

The data is then entered into computer software (within no more than seven days including the day of admission). Home care Resource Groups (HHRGs) for clinical factors, functional factors, and service utilization factors for Medicare recipients will be scored from the responses to the OASIS indicator items (or triggers) to determine the amount of money the agency will receive for providing care for the client (Sienkiewicz & Narayan, 2002). Insurance company case managers, who may be non-nurses, determine disciplines and frequencies or number of visits. They usually require the documentation of each visit faxed to them for a continuous review of the need for home care services and to review outcomes of the care received. Assessment data for both privately insured and private-pay clients are entered into the agency's information system within the agency's mandated timeframe.

The computer software generates the plan of care on the standardized form (HCFA-485). This form is sent to the physician for signature certifying that the client does have a medical condition and requires the skilled care written on the HCFA-485. The **certification,** once signed by the physician, is the order for the care of that client by home care providers. The plan of care contains demographic data, medications, treatments, diet, allergies, disciplines and their frequencies and orders, supplies or medical equipment, expected outcomes, and prognosis. The plan of care is then mailed or hand-carried to the physician's office for his or her review and signature. The client is thus "certified" to receive home care and services for 60 days (Centers for Medicare & Medicaid Services, 2005).

The plan of care is dynamic and can be amended constantly according to the client's health status and needs during the 60-day period. Additional physician's orders written during that 60-day certification period supersede the original orders. The physician's orders received must be carefully documented and filed in the client's chart to justify any change made to the plan of care. The nurse who receives the order is responsible for writing the order and communicating the new order to the primary nurse or therapist and if necessary, the client. If the primary nurse or therapist obtained the order, he or she is responsible for documenting the order and communicating with appropriate personnel and the client. The orders are usually verbal telephone orders. Therefore, the original is placed in each individual physician's folder and is mailed or hand-carried to the physician for signature. A copy is placed on the client's chart in the agency office until the signed order is returned.

A new HCFA-485 or plan of care is required for each 60-day certification. After the initial 60-day certification period the client will be discharged from home care if there is no longer a need for skilled care. The client may receive another comprehensive assessment just days prior to the end of the certification and skilled care may need to continue for another 60-day period. This time period and any other 60-day periods until discharged from home care are called recertification (USDHHS: HCFA, 2000).

A comprehensive assessment and a new set of physician's orders are also required for the client if there is an acute care, skilled care, or rehabilitation (inclient) stay. This assessment is referred to as a post-hospital assessment or with the advent of OASIS, resumption of care (ROC). If there is a significant change in condition (SCIC), a major decline or improvement in health status, a comprehensive assessment is completed. The assessments for those clients discharged from inclient stays are completed within 24 hours after the home care agency is notified they have been discharged. The SCIC is conducted as soon as the need is recognized by the health care provider. The forms for the time periods are agency-specific; but all have integrated the OASIS data set indicators that will affect Medicare PPS reimbursement. The new set of orders that result will supersede the HCFA-485 plan of care completed for the initial start of care or recertification. Disciplines and frequency of visits may change as a result of any of the assessments previously mentioned (USDHHS: HCFA, 2000).

Coordination of Services

Coordination of the multidiscipline team is an essential component of assisting the client make a smooth transition from acute care to home care or for the provision of efficient, cost-effective, quality home care delivery. Although each discipline visits the client separately, the plan of care developed by the client/caregiver, nurse or therapist, and physician dictates the frequency of those visits, the skills each discipline is to provide, and the desired client outcome. The coordination of the client's care begins when the referral to evaluate the client for admission is received.

Some home care agencies assign an RN or LPN/LVN whose primary responsibility is to take the referrals and an RN to serve as a liaison between the home care agency and the acute care or long-term care facilities' discharge managers. It is important to note that it is unethical and illegal for the home care coordinator to visit the client or to have any other contact with the client until the client has made the definitive choice of that particular agency (Zuber, 2001). Other home care agencies delegate the intake of referrals and coordination of care to the nurse manager, case manager, or team leader. Large home care agencies may employ a coordinator of professional services and a coordinator of home care aide services. Regardless of the system used, the coordinators who assist the professional nurses and therapists are registered nurses who have home care nursing experience; leadership skills; organizational, critical-thinking, and decision-making skills; are knowledgeable about home care policies and procedures; and have an understanding of reimbursement guidelines. The home care aide coordinator may be a clerical worker who has demonstrated organizational and leadership skills, knowledge about home care policies and procedures, as well as critical-thinking and decision-making skills regarding schedules, making efficient and cost-effective assignments based on geographical location, required skills, and reimbursement guidelines for frequencies. Both the professional and the aide coordinator must possess effective verbal and written communication skills and possess a customer service orientation.

Some agencies assign RNs a client caseload in the same general geographical area that they coordinate and manage daily. The caseload provides a minimum of visits per week (agency-specific requirement). The nurse calls into the office or voicemail reporting the sequence of visits planned each morning. Any changes in the schedule are communicated with the coordinator. The nurse might need to change a daily schedule to accommodate another schedule or a client's request, or if a client has a change in condition or new orders are received. When these events occur, the coordinator informs the nurse via voicemail, pager, or cell phone during the day. Other agencies assign the same clients to the same nurse the majority of the time, but the team leader or coordinator manages the schedule and maintains control of the number of visits per nurse each week. The coordinator informs the nurse each afternoon about the following day's visit schedule. The nurse calls in the sequence of clients the following morning and is informed of any changes. These are two common types of daily coordination of home care visits, but this may differ in each home care agency.

The RN plans each day's visits according to the most cost-effective route, that is, with no "doubling back and forth" between clients. Generally, it is easier to travel in a circle from the closest client as the starting point and end with the client nearest the office or the nurse's home. The sequence may need to be adjusted more than once during the day if a client requires an unexpected visit because of a change in health status and/or a physician's order, if another nurse requires assistance with visits, or supervised aide visits need to be coordinated. The nurse is notified by the coordinator when a client on the nurse's schedule is being discharged from the hospital or of new admissions to be conducted the following day.

The social worker or nurse in an inclient facility notifies the home care agency when a home care client is to be discharged and the post-hospital or resumption of care (ROC) visit is scheduled for the following day. If the client is a new referral, the nurse who manages a client caseload in the same geographical area in which the new client resides will be assigned the initial comprehensive assessment the day following receipt of the referral. If the nurse's schedule cannot be arranged to accommodate the comprehensive assessment, another nurse may perform the initial assessment. Clients who have special needs or complex health problems may have a physician's order for the nurse to visit the same day of discharge.

The RN coordinator, team leader, or case manager also maintains the therapists' schedules, but the therapists set the frequencies and they basically manage their individual schedules. The coordinator, however, is responsible for communicating to therapists any new referrals or that clients need a post-hospital visit, notifying them of any changes in orders received, and for frequency compliance with physician orders. Therapists may have clients in several geographical areas and may schedule visits, when possible, on certain days by area. The RN coordinator is also responsible for nurses' and therapists' travel audits and their performance appraisals. Additionally, the RN coordinator assists in the interview process for hiring; monitors compliance with all policies, procedures, and reimbursement guidelines; and assists with staff development.

The home care aides are usually assigned clients within a circumscribed geographical area similar to the RNs. However, the aide may see clients from several nurses' schedules. Supervised aide visits are coordinated between the nurse and the aide or by the coordinators. The primary RN and the coordinators are responsible for the bimonthly supervision (supervised and unsupervised visits) compliance for all clients who receive the assistance of a home care aide.

The home care aide coordinator develops each aide's schedule based on the frequency of visits ordered for each client, client preferences for days of the week and times of the day, and geographic location. In agencies that have both the RN and aide coordinators, they collaborate to make certain the nurses and aides are compliant with the required number of supervised and unsupervised visits. The aide coordinator, like the RN coordinator, is responsible for travel audits, performance appraisals, staff development, and fielding phone calls from clients and care providers during the day. Aide coordinators use the same systems of communication with the home care aides as the RN coordinators use with the nurses.

The redesigning, reengineering, and restructuring of home care agencies required with the advent of the PPS has resulted in fewer staff and health care providers to coordinate the same or a higher volume of work. Some agencies may assign one nurse to coordinate all of the health care providers and the schedules as described above. The fact that the responses to the OASIS items help determine the amount of reimbursement for Medicare clients has increased the need for coordination and continued guidance so that the agency is reimbursed correctly for the care and services provided.

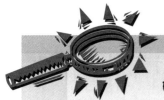

Evidence-Based Practice Box 2-1

Coordination of Services and Evidence-Based Practice Improve Health Status for Heart Failure Clients

Health care professionals at a large health care system in Wisconsin sought to improve the home status of heart failure (HF) clients under their care, thereby decreasing the number of hospital readmissions and shortening the lengths of stay. The group accomplished their goals by combining coordinated efforts across their system of hospitals, clinics, home care, and hospices, and adapting evidence-based practices for HF. Practice guidelines were established using the American Heart Association Guidelines for HF management.

Practitioners were divided into four groups: research and data collection, client education, telephone follow-up, and implementation. Implementation was started at the acute care sites and progressed to home care. Clients were followed at 30-day and 90-day intervals.

System-wide outcomes included an increase in prescription and use of appropriate cardiac medications, decrease in readmission rates, and shorter lengths of stay when readmitted.

(Miranda et al., 2002)

Interdisciplinary team collaboration and conferences are an essential component of the coordination of home care and services. Formal meetings, memos, progress notes, and phone calls are methods for the disciplines to communicate on a continuous basis. This is particularly true when a client returns from a hospitalization or rehabilitation, is to be recertified, or has a change in social or health status. The primary concerns of each discipline and the coordination of care are to assure the delivery of cost-effective quality home care that will result in quality client outcomes.

Outcomes and Assessment Information Set (OASIS)

OASIS is a group of uniform data sets designed to evaluate the consistency and quality of care provided and to quantify the outcomes of home care. A client outcome is defined as a change in health status between two timepoints while the client receives home care services (for example, the time between the start of care and discharge). OASIS was developed over a 12-year period of collaboration between the Centers for Medicare and Medicaid Services (CMS) and the Robert Wood Johnson Foundation at the Center for Health Services Research, Denver. A study was initiated to develop a system of outcome measures for home care to fulfill the provisions of the Balanced Budget Act (BBA) of 1997 that provided for prospective payment. This provision of the BBA became effective in October 2000 and the last revision was October 1, 2002. The resulting OASIS has made it possible to provide states with the information to direct onsite home care agency inspections, generate agency-level case mix reports that contain aggregate statistics on client characteristics at the standardized timepoints, provide a quality improvement system for internal performance improvement, and provide a centralized database to compare quality and outcomes on a national level (Centers for Medicare & Medicaid Services, 2005).

The OASIS set consists of 82 specific questions that must be answered by the home care agency. Each question has a specific code number. Examples of these codes would be MO390 "Vision with corrective lenses" if the patient usually wears them, or MO700 "Ambulation/ Locomotion." There are standardized timepoints for data collection for adult clients over 18 years of age. OASIS is not used for clients under age 18 or prenatal clients. The timepoints are at the start of care, transfer to an acute care facility, resumption of care following an inclient stay, recertification or every 60 days following the start of care but not earlier than 5 days before the end of the certification period, and a significant change in condition (SCIC), which can be a decline or improvement in health status, discharge, or death (Community Health Accreditation Program, 2002; Centers for Medicare & Medicaid Services, 2005).

OASIS questions are also called outcome indicators, triggers, or case-mix indicators. The items encompass sociodemographic, environmental, support system, health status, and functional status as well as selected attributes of health service utilization. The responses to these items by the person conducting these assessments determine the clinical status, functional status, and the utilization (services needed) at the time of data collection. The OASIS measures client acuity as well as outcomes; thus the items predict care needs and costs before care is provided. These items, congruent with Medicare Home Care Conditions of Participation (COP), are directly related to PPS and all Medicare-certified home care agencies are required by CMS to integrate the OASIS data collection into each assessment at the standardized timepoints (Centers for Medicare & Medicaid Services, 2005; OASIS Education and Training, 1999).

The OASIS data set cannot stand alone as a comprehensive or complete assessment. Medicare and Medicaid mandate that OASIS be integrated into all Medicare-certified home care agency standardized assessment timepoints. The forms may not be consistent across agencies, but the OASIS data required is included in each agency's forms. For example, each agency may generate its own forms for a discharge visit, start of care, or transfer to another agency. Regardless of the agency or forms used, they must contain the OASIS PPS indicators. These indicators impact the amount the agency will be paid for providing the care to the client and are highlighted on each form.

OASIS data collection at the start of care is done by the RN or PT assigned to evaluate/ admit the client. OASIS data collection for the other timepoints is done by the primary nurse or therapist. The last professional health care provider who sees the client completes the discharge OASIS (USDHHS: HCFA, 1999). OASIS data is entered into software specifically designed to assign Home Care Resource Group (HHRG) scores to the three domains of data collected: clinical, functional, and service utilization. Each of these domains have specific MO questions that are used to calculate a case mix number that determines the actual dollar amount the agency will be reimbursed to provide care for that client. The amount may be increased or decreased during the certification period depending on the assessments completed during that time period. For example, if there is a SCIC and the health status of a client becomes more complex, the agency PPS may increase. The information is then electronically transmitted to the state system, which collects OASIS data in accordance with CMS specifications.

The OASIS is the cornerstone of the home care PPS. It is used to assist agencies with cost containment, quality improvement systems, and has placed emphasis on evidence-based practice and outcome management in home care. The accuracy of data collection and efficiently meeting timeframes and management of services are critical to a home care agency's survival.

The Home Care Nurse Visit

Enhancement of the continuum of care from acute care facilities to home is a goal shared by a variety of settings and disciplines. Continuity of care involves assisting clients to remain in the home and have available resources that are needed and are responsive to their needs. To ensure that a continuum of care exists, this section will discuss the role of the home care nurse and strategies that the home care nurse can use to assist the client to overcome challenges and remain in the home environment.

Conducting the Home Care Nurse Visit

As previously discussed, the home care nurse visits clients for several purposes. Visits include the comprehensive assessment at the start of care, the supervised and unsupervised home care aides' visits, regular visits to implement the plan of care, reassessment visits for clients following inclient stays and for significant changes in status, and visits to discharge the client from home care services. Regardless of the purpose of the visit, the following guidelines are presented for conducting the visit.

Organizing the Visit

Sometimes getting to the client is half the work. Time at each home, the distance between visits, and the traffic must all be considered if a reasonable schedule is to be maintained. Not having everything necessary for client care on arrival can cause overwhelming frustration. Prior to starting the day, home care nurses need to review their client schedules and purposes of the visits. The nurse must organize the schedule in a manner that is considerate of the clients' preferences for time of visit if possible, and is feasible and efficient in terms of time and travel. A phone call to the client's home to verify the time and purpose for the visit may be helpful, especially if the family is supposed to obtain supplies, medications, or equipment needed for the visit.

Safety

Each specialty in nursing has its own brand of stress, and home care is no exception. The nurse is somewhat less safe in the home care setting than in an acute care environment. Automobile time, exposure to neighborhood danger, and lack of proper equipment increase the chances for accidents. Other unsafe conditions include aggressive pets, an unsafe home environment, and difficult and/or violent clients or family members. An important step in the prevention of unsafe conditions is obtaining information from the client and family over the phone when the first home visit is scheduled. The nurse can communicate the expectation to the client for a safe work environment. Asking the client if there are any pets in the home and how they will be managed during the visit can save problems. The nurse can inquire if there are any difficult relationships with family members or neighbors. During the home visit the nurse should not hesitate to establish steps to establish a safe environment, or to exit an environment and notify the supervisor until its safety has been secured.

Assessment

The home care nurse performs the initial comprehensive assessment that will serve as a baseline for future assessments. Client/caregiver preferences for days and times of visits, specific entrances into the client's home to be used by health care providers, or safety information should be obtained on this initial visit. The nurse obtains the client's signature on any documents required by the agency. Such documents include, but are not limited to, a consent form for treatment, schedule of discipline visits planned, and a confidentiality statement. Information about advanced directives and the client's bill of rights are explained to the client. These forms are signed by both the nurse and the client.

Table 2-1 summarizes the basic components of the home care nurse visit assessment. The nurse needs to establish rapport with the client and family during the first visit. Avoidance of nursing jargon assists clients and families to understand the nurse and their plans of care. It is important that the home care nurse is aware of and sensitive to the cultural beliefs and practices that may affect the client's health or illness (Andrews and Boyle, 2003; Leininger, 2002). Refer to the evidenced-based practice box in Chapter 3 for an example of implementing cultural practices into a client's plan of care.

The home care nurse is really a visitor in a client's home. Whereas the nurse is in power in acute care settings, the client and the client's caregivers are in power in the home. The client's home is his or her intimate and personal environment, and it is easy for attachment or closeness to develop among the client, the family, and the nurse. The nature of the nurse–client relationship

TABLE 2-1 The Home Care Nurse Assessment	
TYPE	**GUIDELINES**
Physical	Current complaints; history of illnesses and surgeries; review of systems; cephalocaudal assessment with vital signs, weight and height.
Psychosocial	Cognitive abilities; affective assessment; family structure and availability, caregiver assessment, social support systems availability; substance use such as alcohol, tobacco, or medications.
Financial	Type of health care coverage; food stamps; income for food and medications; request to see all insurance cards, if home care instituted after an accident, describe the accident.
Environment	Home structure and modifications; fall risks; sanitation; neighborhood for safety and support.
Nutrition	Type of diet; if noncompliant, describe why; appetite; 24-hour diet recall; food preparation and responsibility; OTC vitamins or dietary supplements.
Functional	Any assistive devices used; ability to perform activities of daily living (ADL) such as dressing, eating, and toileting; and speech pattern difficulties.
Community	Transportation; access to health care; participation in senior center activities, support groups; any neighbors or friends involved in care regularly.

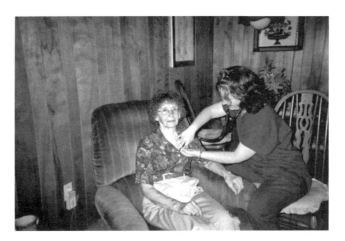

Figure 2-1 Jackie Magelssen, RN, BSN, conducts the admission assessment for a home care client.

is time limited; therefore plans for termination of the relationship begin with the first visit. The nurse should focus on assisting the client and family to attain positive outcomes and establish professional and personal boundaries. These boundaries may be flexible, but there needs to be a strong sense of the nurse–client relationship from the initial encounter (Durkin, 2000).

Each successive regular visit should include inquiries about signs and symptoms, the effectiveness of treatments, appetite and nutrition, any doctor visits that have occurred since the last home care visit, any changes made in medications, or if any new problems have arisen. These queries may cue the client to provide information previously forgotten that might require follow-up or closer scrutiny.

Generally the nurse starts the physical assessment by taking vital signs and weight, and uses a cephalocaudal sequence to conduct the physical examination at each regular visit (Figure 2-1). The type of visit may also affect the assessment. While the regular visits routinely monitor the effectiveness of care and outcomes management, the recertification assessment is conducted to discern the need for further skilled care as well as outcomes.

The resumption of care (ROC), also referred to as a post-inclient stay assessment, can follow acute care, skilled care, or rehabilitation stays. A comprehensive assessment is required that includes the OASIS items to indicate changes in clinical or functional status or service utilization following inclient care. An unanticipated change in the health status of the client (SCIC) requires a comprehensive assessment and the OASIS items may trigger a reduced payment or an increased payment for the agency.

Implementation of Procedures/Treatments

The plan of care will specify procedures and treatments that the home care nurse must implement. The physician orders specify the frequency and specifics regarding the treatment required. Client condition, environmental setting, and other variables may prompt the nurse to modify how the procedure is done. When modifications are made, adherence to standards of practice and standard precautions must be maintained. Throughout the procedure the nurse should assess and evaluate the client, and modify the intervention as needed to maintain client safety and security. Client teaching should be routinely incorporated during the procedure.

Adaptability is one of the key skills needed by the home care nurse in carrying out procedures and treatments in the home. Lack of space, unfamiliar supplies/equipment, and lack of convenient articles such as IV poles, convenient electrical outlets, close proximity to water and disposal sources forces the need to be creative. Examples of creativity may be the need to use a trouble light for additional lighting or a floor lamp as an IV pole.

Monitoring Medication Therapy

Comprehensive medication reviews are usually done on admission, at the time of discharge, after hospitalization, and at any time there is a new medication prescribed. The following guidelines for monitoring medication therapy are presented:

- Before the client visit, the nurse should review all of the records available.
- During the visit, the nurse should state the purpose for this interview and ask the client what medications the physicians have prescribed. For each medication, the nurse should ask the following:
  - Why are you taking this medication?
  - How long have you been taking this medication?
  - How do you take this medication (dosage, frequency)?
  - How does this medication help your problem?
  - Do you take any over-the-counter medications?
  - What medications?
  - How often do you take them?
  - What do you take them for?
  - Do they help?

The nurse should assess the client's knowledge of the medication regimen and the client's compliance with the prescribed regimen. The client should be able to state the purpose of the medication, the correct dose, and the sequence for taking the medication. The nurse should assess any problems caused by the medication including adverse effects, financial problems, or treatment failures. The nurse will list on each assessment form and nurses' note the current prescribed medications, their dosages, and their administration schedules. The frequency of recoding this list is agency specific. The nurse should summarize the client's management system and the client's ability to follow directions and his or her level of compliance with the prescribed medication regime.

Teaching

The nurse will need to develop a plan to correct any problems uncovered during the interview. Client teaching should be routinely incorporated into every home nurse visit. Client education is essential in promoting personal health responsibility and compliance. Education should be considered a routine part of most interventions. Informed clients are often less anxious, more cooperative, provide better histories, and are more proactive regarding their health care.

The home care nurse must be sensitive and able to accommodate teaching style to meet the needs of the client and primary caregiver. For example, elder clients may require creative communication skills due to difficulty hearing or understanding. The nurse must be careful in level of language and choice of words to enable the client with low literacy to be able to comprehend the information. The nurse must ascertain who else needs the information, so that the primary caregiver as well as the client both have the information needed for them to perform self-care. Refer to Chapter 3 for a more in-depth discussion of client teaching.

Documentation

The accurate collection of data and subsequent documentation of assessments can make the difference in outcome measurement and, ultimately, the amount of reimbursement an agency receives from third-party payers. The documentation must accurately reflect the acuity of the client, the functional abilities of the client, the results of assessments, any treatments/procedures performed and the client's response, information about the caregiver's ability to meet the client's home care needs, and the client/caregiver's knowledge deficits. If information is reported to the physician, the pharmacist is called for refills, or any other communication occurs during the visit, the nurse should document the communication in the nurse's notes. The nurse should document in the nurse's note any plans to communicate with other professionals following the visit.

Accurate documentation of the nurse's arrival and departure time for each visit cannot be overemphasized. The manipulation or falsification of times of visits or information regarding visits is considered fraudulent behavior and can result in legal action against the perpetrator. The nurse's documentation of each visit should reflect the client's progress toward meeting the outcome goals of care established in the plan of care. If the goals remain unmet, this should be documented along with a revised plan of care. It is essential to remember that the chart is a documentation of what was done, as well as a legal record. The record also provides a means of communication between disciplines, the administration, and the payer sources. The adage of "if it's not written, it's not done" is just as important in home care as it is in acute care because documentation can affect a home care client's care and the agency's financial viability.

Medications and the Elderly

Every home care nurse's visit includes monitoring his or her clients' use and misuse of medications. It has become increasingly apparent that the management of aging clients differs from the management of younger clients. One key factor in understanding adverse medication reactions in the elderly is to understand the changes which age itself brings. On one level, more medications are taken as a response to more ailments, especially chronic diseases. On another level there is a change in the physiology of the aged that influences the pharmacology of the medications administered to them. The following physiological changes alter the way medications operate in the elderly and suggest that the aged are at greater risk for medication toxicity (Running and Berndt, 2003):

- *Absorption.*   The gastrointestinal tract function is slowed, resulting in less complete medication absorption.
- *Distribution.*   The cardiovascular system is often sluggish, causing decreased or delayed medication circulation. Body composition changes, with a decrease in the amount of total body water and in the percentage of body weight that is water. This can result in a decrease in the volume and distribution of medications that are distributed in body water and an increase in volume for fat-soluble medications.
- *Metabolism.*   Studies suggest that the metabolizing capability of liver enzymes decreases with age. There is a decrease in liver blood flow with age affecting the metabolism of some medications.
- *Excretion.*   Glomerular filtration rate, creatinine clearance, and renal blood flow all decrease with age. These changes can result in a decreased excretion of medications from the body.

There are a number of indicators to suggest that medication problems increase in both number and seriousness with the elderly. Unfortunately, many adverse medication reactions go unrecognized. New signs and symptoms may be attributed to acute or chronic illness rather than to a change in medication therapy. One of the most important contributions that the home care nurse can make to an older person's well-being is to have a high index of suspicion about adverse medication reactions. There is less chance of missing adverse medication effects if one automatically questions if a new symptom could be due to medication therapy.

Medication Use and Misuse

Elderly persons who are managing their own medications frequently misuse medications in one or more ways (Box 2-1).

Some typical causes of problems with medications are as follows:

- *Sharing medications*. Elders often share medications in an attempt to help out a friend by providing something that has helped them and save the cost of a doctor's visit.
- *Hoarding medications*. Elders may use medications that have been prescribed at an earlier time. The risks associated with this are inaccurate self-diagnosis or self-treatment, and the use of outdated medications.
- *Self-medication*. Elders often medicate themselves with nonprescription medications, vitamins, herbs, or home remedies. These practices are not necessarily harmful, but may prevent the elder from seeking needed medical evaluation and can cause interactive adverse effects with other medications.
- *Duplicate medications*. Elders often are seen by multiple physicians and do not inform them of all the medications that they are taking. With the use of more generic brands of medications, consumers can easily have medications that are different in color, size, and shape yet are the same medication.
- *Noncompliance.* There are a number of reasons elders are more likely to be noncompliant than younger people. Some of these reasons include:
  - *Lack of understanding.* The elder client or primary caregiver may not understand the purpose or action of a medication and will attempt to set up a medication system based on their own understanding. This problem is particularly likely when there are frequent medication changes, or unclear instructions such as "take as directed."
  - *Adverse medication reactions.* Adverse medication reactions may cause an elder to stop taking a medication or decrease the dose.
  - *Cost.* The cost of medications is a major factor in compliance because for many elders on a fixed income medications are a large part of their monthly budget.

BOX 2-1 TYPICAL ERRORS IN SELF-ADMINISTRATION OF MEDICATIONS

- Omission or failure to take a prescribed medication
- Incorrect dosage
- Improper time or sequence
- Inaccurate knowledge

They often omit doses to try to stretch out a prescription, may delay in getting a prescription filled, or simply not have the prescription filled in the first place.

- *Memory deficits*. As individuals age there is some loss of short-term memory function. When taking multiple medications at multiple times it is often hard for the elder to remember if he or she has taken a previous dose.
- *Physical limitations*. Some people are physically limited to comply with their medication regimen due to poor vision, inability to swallow medications, or decreased strength to open containers. Mobility problems may limit access to pharmacies or the ability to refill medications prior to running out.

Guidelines for Enhancing Compliance

The home care nurse can play an essential role in assisting the elder and primary caregiver to enhance compliance with their medication regimen. The following guidelines are suggested:

- *Perform an assessment*. Assess the elder and caregiver's understanding of medications and reasons/rationale that they may not comply or adhere to the regime.
- *Promote understanding*. The nurse must offer information in language and manner appropriate to the person. The nurse needs to validate understanding of the elder or primary caregiver and reinstruct as needed.
- *Be alert for adverse medication effects*. Encourage elders to inform the health care provider if they think there are any untoward signs or symptoms. The nurse needs to be especially observant when new medications are added or dosages are changed.
- *Simplify the regimen*. Work with the elder's daily schedule to determine a convenient pattern for taking medications.
- *Introduce memory aids*. Assist the elder to develop a system to remember medications. A variety of medi-planners are available at pharmacies. These containers enable the elder or caregiver to fill the box for a week at a time, as the box has compartments for different dosing times. Egg carton containers, small plastic bags, or plastic wrap can be used to hold the day's supply of medications. Placing the medications next to a calendar can assist the elder to write down the medication and dose every time it is taken.
- *Manage physical barriers*. Suggest that the elder purchase non-childproof caps for containers if there is difficulty in opening them.
- *Decrease medication costs*. Encourage the elder to discuss cost concerns with their prescriber. This will encourage the prescriber to use generic medications that may be cheaper or to provide samples of new medications before a prescription is filled.

Assisting elders with safe medication administration is one of the most important tasks that the home care nurse faces daily. It is vitally important that the client understand the medication; its effects; side effects; and drug, food, and over-the-counter medication interactions.

Working with Clients' Caregivers

Caregiving is a reality for most Americans. Until recently, most health problems and care were dealt with by professionals. Today, it is estimated that 44.4 million people in the United States are unpaid caregivers to individuals and their family members (Panda, 2005). Home care services can lessen the burden of lay caregivers, but they cannot assume the role of the primary caregiver. The caregiver plays a major role in the health care delivery system and it is up to the home care nurse to empower care recipients and/or caregivers to assume responsibility for their health and health care. Empowerment requires that the home care nurse identify health risk factors and intervene so that primary caregivers receive the support they need in order to care for those who depend on them.

The responsibility and obligation for the caregiving role of families is fraught with problems, and the quality of care provided may be impacted by these caregiving problems. The family may be the client's best support system and the role of the nurse is one of educator, advocate, and facilitator. In other cases, when the family is absent or refuses to comply with instructions, the home care nurse must problem-solve to find other alternatives to ensure quality long-term care for the recipient. This section will discuss symptoms of stress that the nurse should assess in caregivers and suggest strategies for dealing with caregiver problems.

Identify High-Risk Areas

Research over the past couple of decades has demonstrated that long-term caregiving for a family member can produce a number of negative consequences, including psychological and emotional strain, physical and financial strain, job conflicts, and family disruption. The home care nurse should take the time to talk with caregivers about their problems and concerns, and to assess for symptoms of caregiver role strain (Box 2-2).

Caregivers need someone who listens and lets them talk about their feelings without being judgmental or giving unwanted advice. Home care nurses are in a good position to do this because they are more objective than family members and friends. The following section discusses assessment cues and ways nurses can assist caregivers to cope with common stressors.

Psychological and Emotional Strain   The effect on family members caring for a physically ill person in the home has been referred to as burden, strain, role fatigue, and caregiver stress (Mignor, 2000). Caregiver well-being is a concern for several reasons. Stress can cause physical and emotional illness in the caregiver, thus creating another client. Stressed caregivers often cannot provide good, safe care. Institutionalization, neglect, abuse, and physical and mental deterioration of the recipient of care have been related to caregivers stress (Brock, 1998). Numerous studies have confirmed that caregivers are at higher risk for depression than the general population (Mignor, 2000). Cues to the caregiver's depression may be complaints of insomnia, weight changes, sadness, brooding, fatigue, and loss of interest in formerly pleasurable activities.

The nurse has a role in helping caregivers to recognize that their feelings and responses to the situation are normal and legitimate. The problems associated with psychological strain can

---

BOX 2-2 SIGNS AND SYMPTOMS OF CAREGIVER ROLE STRAIN

Physical: headaches, fatigue, loss of appetite, hypertension

Emotional: anger, sadness, anxiety, guilt, loneliness, hopelessness

Cognitive: forgetfulness, difficulty making decisions, inability to concentrate

Interpersonal: blaming others, impatience, withdrawal

Spiritual: loss of life satisfaction, feelings of alienation

be relieved by planned periods of respite. The nurse can assist the caregiver to identify individuals who would be willing to provide time to sit with the care recipient to enable the primary caregiver to get out of the house or at least have some time free of the recipient. Developing a formal schedule with other family members to relieve the caregiver and to provide elements of care for periods of time—such as evenings, a couple hours in the afternoon, or weekends—is effective. Some churches or social groups have volunteers who are available to stay with a person for several hours. Other options include having homemakers, retired persons, or high school or college students to provide relief. Referring caregivers to community-based caregiver support groups or Internet sites for caregivers are other options.

Physical Strain Caregiving can be physically stressful. Caregiving tasks often require frequent bending, lifting, and moving. Additionally, psychological stress can contribute to stress-related physical problems. Many caregivers do not see to their own health care needs on a regular basis, and often delay seeking treatment for their own health problems (Mignor, 2000). Changes in physical health may be related to caregivers' lack of time or energy to engage in health-promoting behaviors such as exercise, good nutrition, or stress management.

Caregivers may need advice about exercise, nutrition, health care, and stress management. The nurse should take time to check the caregiver's BP or weight, or inquire about their medications and give them an opportunity to talk about problems and concerns. Suggestions to the caregiver to help relieve caregiver stress may include:

- Sharing the responsibility for care.
- Taking on only what can be handled.
- Involving others who can help out.
- Meditating and listening to music.
- Engaging in mild exercise like walking.

Caregivers who do not take care of themselves will burn out and be of no use to anyone.

Set Priorities

Setting priorities is one way to decrease caregiver strain. Suggestions for setting priorities include:

- Working on one problem at a time.
- Maintaining physical health by taking time for oneself, eating right, avoiding medications and alcohol, and getting regular exercise.
- Seeking the help of others such as family, clergy, and friends.
- Learning about caregiving.
- Joining support groups.
- Learning about available resources in the community.

Educate the Caregiver

The major goals of caregiver education should be to empower the caregiver and to increase caregiver competence. The following strategies are helpful:

- Help caregivers set goals and expectations.
- Educate the caregiver to provide needed skills.
- Help caregivers solve problems.

Caregivers are more likely to do something if they believe they can be successful. Therefore, the goal of education should be to provide the caregivers with the confidence that they can do a task. This means providing the caregiver with the opportunity to practice skills.

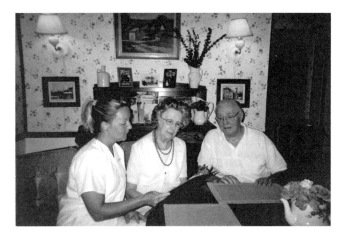

Figure 2-2 An RN reviews the plan of care with a client and his caregiver.

Contrary to the myth that the ill and infirm are abandoned by their families, the family is often the client's strongest social support and the major provider of health care services. Family caregivers are responsible for providing supportive services, personal care, and often complex skilled health care services to the community-dwelling individual. The success of this role is largely contingent on the assessment and supervision of the home care nurse (Figure 2-2).

Discharge Planning

An essential component of the concept of continuity of care is discharge planning. The purpose of discharge planning is to move a client from one health care delivery setting to another, or to self-care in a manner that assures quality client outcomes and facilitates continuity of care. This purpose can only be met by the cooperative efforts of all parties involved. This cooperation includes the professionals, para-professionals, support persons, the client, and the client's family. Emphasis is on communication, education, collaboration, and cooperation.

Continuity of Care

The emphasis in health care over the last few decades has been toward cost containment via offering high-quality care in a time-effective, cost-effective manner across the continuum of care. To achieve this goal, discharge planning has become an essential and continuous process in assessing client needs and developing an appropriate cost-effective plan of care to facilitate the movement of the client to the most appropriate setting (Zuber, 2001).

Figure 2-3 depicts the continuum of care to be accomplished through good discharge planning. The model implies that clients can enter the formal health care delivery system through a variety of settings, including the emergency room, their primary care provider, an ambulatory care setting, or hospital. It is essential for discharge planning to begin at the point of entry to assess client needs and facilitate the client into most appropriate cost-effective setting. The model also depicts that movement through the continuum of care may be multidirectional as indicated by the arrows. The arrows demonstrate that the client's needs can change, and as they change, movement to a more appropriate setting may be indicated. Skills in discharge planning are essential to assure that the client is appropriately placed within the continuum of care.

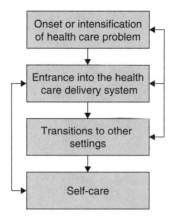

Figure 2-3 Continuum of care

Use of the Nursing Process in Discharge Planning

Discharge planning from home care should be incorporated into the components of the nursing process. These components include assessment, nursing diagnoses, planning, implementation, and evaluation. This section will discuss the unique skills that the home care nurse needs to use in applying the nursing process to discharge planning.

Assessment   The objectives of assessment include:

- Identify the care and services of a home care agency including disciplines and services offered, coordination of care, plan of treatment, and care outcomes.
- Describe the purpose and components of the home care nurse visit.
- Understand and identify strategies to assess and enhance the challenges the home care nurse encounters in delivering care.
- Discuss the process of discharge planning.

   Discharge planning begins the day the client is admitted to the agency. The nurse needs to assess the specific learning needs, the client's and family's perceptions of outcomes, financial needs, and the human and materials supports/resources required by the client. Consultation with other health care providers is an essential part of the comprehensive assessment for discharge planning.

Nursing Diagnosis   The assessment data will determine the nursing diagnoses that are needed for discharge planning. For example, the nurse may determine that there is a knowledge deficit, caregiver strain, or ineffective management of the therapeutic regimen. It is extremely important that there is documentation and communication of the nursing diagnoses to all members of the team. This ensures that members are not working at cross-purposes to one another.

Planning   Planning begins with writing and communicating client oriented outcomes of care. The outcomes should identify what is expected in measurable behavioral terms including the goals, strategies to accomplish the goals, specific outcomes, and indices to measure achievement.

Implementation   Interventions reflect the strategies used specific to each goal established in the planning process. The nurse selects and prioritizes appropriate activities that will lead to the achievement of each expected outcome. The primary care nurse is responsible for the selection, implementation, and documentation of the specific activities used with each client.

Evaluation   Every visit with the client must evaluate the client's progress in meeting the expected health care outcomes. A thorough evaluation will identify strengths and weaknesses in the care plan. The evaluation will determine if the goals of the client have been achieved or if the plan of care should be modified. It is essential that the nurse document, communicate, and coordinate with all team members the evaluative data. The evaluative data will determine when the client's goals have been met, and then planning for transition to another setting, professional care, or self-care will result.

Humphrey and Milone-Nuzzo (1996) identified criteria for discharging a client from home care. These criteria include achievement of goals as initially determined, ceased needing skilled nursing care or therapy, hospitalization, refusal of care, relocation of the client outside the agency's service area, and/or death of the client.

At the time of discharge from home health, the nurse needs to document on the discharge form the reason for discharge, summarize the care given, describe the way goals were met, and describe the client's status at the time of discharge. This information should be communicated to the client's primary provider as well as to the setting the client is being transitioned to if applicable. The client should receive, in writing, notification of discharge, instructions for continued care, and specifics as to who to contact for referrals or in case of a problem.

Summary

Home care can be defined as the provision of services, education, and a setting for the purpose of maintaining or restoring a client's maximum level of health, function, and comfort. The key to achieving these goals is to coordinate all of the services available to the client.

This chapter identified the various disciplines available through home health, their roles, and how these various providers coordinate the delivery of care in an efficient and effective manner to enable the client to achieve quality health care outcomes and to remain in the community. OASIS, as a system required by Medicare and Medicaid to assure best practice, assess clinical outcomes, and assist agencies with cost containment, was described. The necessity of discharge planning to maximize independence of the client and assure continuity of care was stressed.

The role of the home care nurse was described with emphasis on the home care visit and the nurse's role as coordinator of care. The section on challenges in caring for clients in the home discussed the importance of the family in home care and special needs of the elder clients with their medications.

References

Andrews, M. M., & Boyle, J. S. (2003). *Transcultural concepts in nursing care.* Philadelphia: Lippincott.

Anemaet, W. K., Krulish, L. H., Lindstrom, K. C., Herr, R., & Carr, M. N. (2001). Evaluating physical therapy utilization under PPS. *Home Healthcare Nurse, 19*(8), 502–505.

Brock, A. M. (1998). Elder caregivers: Their challenges, trails, and triumphs. *Nursing Connections, 11*(2), 18–23.

Brown, J., Hasselkus, A., & Tenenholtz, E. (2002). Speech-language pathologists add value to home care. *Home Healthcare Nurse, 20*(6), 393–398.

Bull, P., & Halligan, Sr. C. M. (2002). Growing your own cna's: It's worth the effort. *Home Healthcare Nurse, 20*(1), 18–21.

Centers for Medicare & Medicaid Services (CMS). (2005).
http://cms.hhs.gov/oasis/oasisdat.asp

Community Health Accreditation Program (CHAP). (2002). *Home care standards of excellence*. New York, NY.

Durkin, N. (2000). The importance of setting boundaries in home care and hospice nursing. *Home Healthcare Nurse, 18*(7), 478–481.

Humphrey, C. J. (2002). The current status of home care nursing practice: Part 2: Operational trends and future challenges. *Home Healthcare Nurse, 20*(11), 741–746.

Humphrey, C. T., & Milone-Nuzzo, P. (1996). *Orientation to home care nursing*. Gaithersburg, MD: Aspen.

Krulish, L. H. (2000). When should I do an OASIS assessment? *Home Healthcare Nurse, 18*(4), 238.

Leininger, M. M. (2002). *Transcultural nursing: Concepts, theories, research, and practice* (3rd ed.). New York: McGraw-Hill.

Mignor, D. (2000). Effectiveness of use of home health nurses to decrease burden & depression of elderly caregivers. *Journal of Psychosocial Nursing, 38*(7), 34–41.

Miranda, M. E., Gorski, L. A., LeFevre, J. G., Levac, K. A., Niederstadt, J. A., & Toy, A. L. (2002). An evidence-based approach to improving care of patients with heart failure across the continuum. *Journal of Nursing Care Quality, 17*(1), 1–4.

Panda, S. M. (April, 2005). *Caregiving in the United States research report*. Washington, DC: AARP.

Running, A., & Berndt, A. (2003). *Management guidelines for nurse practitioners: Working in family practice*. Philadelphia: F. A. Davis Co.

Sienkiewicz, J., & Narayan, M. C. (2002). Have you mastered PPS? *Home Healthcare Nurse, 20*(5), 308–317.

U.S. Department of Health and Human Services: Health Care Financing Administration (USD-HHS: HCFA). (1999). Rules and regulations. *Federal Register, 64*(15), 3747–3763.

U.S. Department of Health and Human Services: Health Care Financing Administration (USD-HHS: HCFA). (2000). PPS final rule. *Federal Register, 65*(128), 41128–41214.

Zuber, R. F. (2001). Home care coordination versus discharge planning: Where is the line. *Home Healthcare Nurse, 19*(10), 652–655.

Chapter 3
Client Education

Deolinda Mignor, RN, DNS

Key Terms

Home Care Nurse-educator	Literacy	Teaching/learning

The role of the nurse as educator is part of nursing in all health delivery settings; however, it is an absolute necessity that the home care nurse be an educator. Education is the vital link between the health care provider, home care client, and plan of care. The need for education related to the client's condition is independent of diagnosis, socioeconomic status, or age. Shorter hospital stays, higher client acuity on discharge from health care facilities, the aging population, and clients' escalating need for knowledge related to their conditions have contributed to the increased importance placed on client teaching and understanding.

The Home Care Nurse-Educator

The **home care nurse-educator** is a registered nurse, employed by a home care agency, who in the course of providing skilled nursing care to clients is teaching the client, caregiver, and family that which they need to know to provide optimal care. The goal of home care education as established by the Joint Commission (JCAHO, 2003) is to provide information in a usable format for the client and caregiver. Client educational activities can be indirect as well as direct. Organizations may be involved in educating other health professionals about providing client education or in developing client education materials and resources used by others. When client education is indirectly provided, the organization is responsible for ensuring that the client education process is implemented and that clients are properly educated.

Teaching/learning can be defined as the process of assessing what is needed to know (by the learner), evaluating the learner's readiness to know, setting learning goals, and providing a mechanism to learn (by the teacher) that ultimately changes behavior. Successful teaching/learning in home care embraces the health care educator, client, caregiver, and family and is based on the expectation of mutual and participatory learning (Box 3-1). To meet this challenge, the nurse-educator is prepared to assess variables that affect the teaching/learning outcome such as the client's physical abilities, educational needs, literacy level, emotional status, home environment including home caregivers and family, and cultural and ethnic background.

"Given the current structure of health care in the United States, nurses, in particular, are responsible for designing and implementing plans and procedures for improving health education and encouraging wellness" (Bastable, 2003, p. 44). To conquer this challenge, the nurse-educator must have a working knowledge of teaching/learning theories. Because the

---

BOX 3-1 JOINT COMMISSION EDUCATION STANDARD

An organization meets the goals of the education standard by educating the client about the following:

- The plan of care, treatment, and services.
- Basic health practices and safety.
- The safe and effective use of medications.
- Nutrition interventions, modified diets, or oral health.
- Safe and effective use of medical equipment or supplies when provided by the organization.
- Understanding pain, the risk for pain, the importance of effective pain management, the pain assessment process and methods for pain management.
- Habilitation and rehabilitation techniques to help clients reach maximum independence possible.
- Personal hygiene and grooming.
- Basic home safety.
- Infection prevention and control.
- Procedures to follow if care, treatment, and services are disrupted by a natural disaster or an emergency.
- Identifying, handling, and disposing of hazardous materials and wastes in a safe and sanitary manner according to law and regulation.
- Storage, handling, and access to medical gases and related supplies. (JCAHO, 2004, p. PC-24).

majority of clients receiving health care in the home are adults, a working knowledge of the principles of adult learning is also necessary. According to the National Association of Home Care (NAHC), of the 7.6 million people who received formal home care services in 1998, 68.6 percent were over the age of 65 (NAHC, 2001).

"Families and clients are making home care the service of choice and the largest consumer group of home care services is the elderly" (Wilson, 2000, p. 113). Some older adults are not able to understand how to maintain their health and when health fails, they are unable to care for themselves. However, an increasing number of older adults are interested in maintaining their health and when necessary, they become interested in their medical conditions, their plans of care, and the factors related to their conditions. It is well known that in the United States there is an increase in the number and proportion of older adults in the general population and there is a corresponding demand for health-related education. One has only to follow the agenda of the American Association of Retired Persons (AARP) to appreciate the level of education, intelligence, and political astuteness that this group of older Americans add to health-related discussions.

There are many teaching/learning theories and approaches available to assist nurse-educators with the educational process of home care clients. Successful teaching/learning results begin with a positive nurse–client relationship and a belief that positive outcomes will follow. The process begins with a basic knowledge of teaching/learning principles and self-education of the nurse, followed by client assessment.

Theories of Learning/Teaching

"Learning involves changing to a new state; it is a state that persists. What can be learned? New thinking strategies, new motor skills, and new attitudes are learned in complex patterns that can promote a new performance" (Redman, 2001, p. 21). Learning theories have existed since early civilizations, with new theories continuing to evolve. Many teaching/learning frameworks have their foundations in the work of the theorists who researched and published their theories in the first half of the 20th century. Learning theories are classified as behavioral theory, formerly called stimulus-response or S-R, and cognitive theory. Social cognitive theory incorporates concepts from both behavioral and cognitive theories. The Theory of *andragogy* (Adult Education) was developed and published by Malcolm Knowles in 1980 (Knowles, 1980; Redman, 2001). Refer to Table 3-1 for a summary of teaching/learning theories.

Adult Learning Theory

Adult learning theory developed and evolved as a necessity to distinguish it from theories of learning that address children. Theories related to the learning and teaching of adults can be traced back to the ancient civilizations of Europe and Asia. The names of early teachers such as Confucius, Plato, Aristotle, Socrates, and Cicero are readily recognized. But not until the early 20th century, with the founding in 1926 of the American Association of Adult Education, did inquiries begin about the unique characteristics of adult learners. By World War II, it was established that "adults could learn and that they possessed interests and abilities that were different from those of children" (Knowles, 1980, pp. 28–29).

In applying Knowles' assumptions to the nurse–client relationship, it is expected that nurse-educators recognize that they are facilitators for their clients' learning. Seeing oneself as a facilitator fosters a sense of partnership and respect between the nurse and client and prevents the client from feelings of inadequacy and insecurity. As Knowles stated, adults are independent learners.

TABLE 3-1 Summary of Teaching/Learning Theories		
THEORY	**PREMISE**	**HEALTH CARE EXAMPLE**
Behavioral Learning/ Stimulus-Response	Organism's response to stimuli may change behavior according to conscquences	The child who cries upon seeing a white lab coat
Behavior Modification	Positive reinforcement (rewards) will change behavior, as will negative reinforcement	Common technique used in professional therapeutic relationships
Cognitive Learning Theory	Cognitive traits such as previous experiences, intellect, and information processing will result in learning	Learning as a result of classroom and clinical experiences
Social Cognitive Theory	Behavior can be positive or negative depending on the model being imitated	Internships, externships, and mentoring programs
Adult Learning Theory	Adult learners are self-directed, arrive at the educational scene with rich experiences, and wish to apply new knowledge immediately	The educator assesses and acknowledges the client's previous experiences and knowledge when developing the teaching/learning plan

Source: Bastable, 2003; Huitt & Hummel, 1997; Knowles, 1980; Townsend, 2000.

The nurse-educator uses adult learning theory when assessing the clients' past experiences, especially those experiences that relate to the current health problem. In addition to clients' personal experiences, many clients and their families now search the Internet for information on health conditions. An educational needs assessment will reveal clients' base of knowledge and understanding of their present plan of care.

The developing learning theory of *gerogogy* concentrates on teaching/learning of the elderly. Although it is generally accepted that adults learn differently from children, some educators have suggested that older adults have their own set of motivators and ways of learning. Research and literature that supports the science of helping older adults learn has been slow in forthcoming (Battershy, 1987).

Teaching/Learning Needs Assessment

Success in implementing a teaching plan requires an in-depth assessment of the client, home, caregiver, and family. Assessment begins with reviewing with the client the condition that has warranted home care. Because preexisting conditions may influence the client's ability to learn, the health assessment incorporates the client's health history. Both the mental and physical status of a client will affect the success of teaching and learning. Medications, both prescribed and over-the-counter, must be documented and evaluated, as adverse effects may affect all systems including mental status, vision, and hearing.

Mental Status

Assessment of the client's mental status is necessary to establish the appropriate level to initiate the teaching/learning process. Mental status includes level of alertness, judgment, intelligence, personality, mood, memory, and attention span. Possible questions that help to establish level of alertness are: Is the client verbally responsive? If the client is not conscious and alert, then the focus of teaching will switch from client to caregiver and family. Does the client speak the same language as the nurse? If not, is there an interpreter in the home? Is the client's response to questions and conversations appropriate? A client who is confused, sedated, or otherwise unable to communicate with the nurse will be limited in responding to teaching/learning possibilities.

"Morale, attitude, and self-esteem tend to be stable throughout the lifespan" (Eliopoulos, 2001, p. 67). Changes in personality (that set of personal characteristics that makes each person an individual) are not expected as a normal consequence of aging. Often what is perceived by others as personality changes in the elderly are the result of physical changes such as skeletal rigidity or decreases in sensory responses. And in assessing the mental status of any client, it is important to remember that education is not synonymous with intellect.

Physical Status

The nurse who admits a client to a home care agency will have completed a comprehensive client physical assessment prior to the development of a personalized plan of care. The nurse-educator, who may or may not be the client's admitting nurse, will use information from the physical assessment as a foundation in developing a teaching plan. Each system of the human body undergoes physical changes with the aging process. Changes that are particularly important to assess in relation to the client's ability to learn new health information are sight, hearing, and coordination. Age-related changes and their negative consequences vary from being barely noticeable to interfering with activities of daily living. Table 3-2 summarizes age-related changes that may interfere with teaching/learning.

Vision   "All knowledge of the world in which we live comes to us through our sensory systems. To survive, we must constantly be aware of the environment and the changes taking place within it" (Saxon & Etten, 2002, p. 125). In the United States, approximately 5.5 million people over the age of 65 are blind or visually impaired (American Foundation for the Blind, 2004). Chronic diseases such as diabetes, glaucoma, and macular degeneration affect vision. But changes in sight also occur merely as a result of growing older. "The most common functional consequences resulting from age-related changes (in vision) include diminished ability to focus on near objects, need for greater illumination, diminished acuity, and narrowing of the visual field" (Miller, 2004, p. 264). The list of activities of daily living that are influenced by decreases in visual acuity is lengthy. Those activities that most affect home care clients in their attempts to learn and understand new information are seeing markers on clocks and reading information on food labels, medication bottles, and health care materials such as handouts and guidelines (Miller, 2004).

During the initial home visit, diminished vision may be easily recognized or the client may offer the information before inquiries are made by the admission nurse. However, the nurse can easily

TABLE 3-2 Age-Related Changes That May Interfere with Teaching/Learning

VISION	INTERVENTION
Decreased visual acuity	Increase illumination. Eliminate glare. Use large print.
Decrease in lightness	Allow extra time for adaptation to light and darkness > 4 minutes.
Increased sensitivity to glare	Reduce exposure to sunlight and bright rooms.
Hearing	
Increased accumulation of cerumen	Routine removal by professional.
Presbycusis	Speak slowly and enunciate clearly.
Interference in perception of high-frequency sounds	Lower pitch of voice. Do not shout. Use touch if appropriate.
Skeletal	
Gradual loss of calcium results in loss of bone strength	Adequate calcium intake.
Changes in cartilage surface result in reduction in flexibility	Exercise, especially walking.
Decrease in strength of tendons/ligaments results in decreased strength and mobility	Physical activity.
Neuromuscular	
Decrease in muscle strength and agility	Exercise regularly.
Dizziness and loss of balance	Change positions slowly.
Decreased reaction time	Allow extra time for activities and avoid activities that require quick reaction time (driving a car).

Source: Jarvis, 2004; Saxon & Etten, 2002.

detect visual problems during the course of the home visit by asking the following questions:

- Does the client have difficulty reading the material contained in teaching handouts?
- Does the client have difficulty with or avoid some of his or her usual activities such as driving, reading, watching television, using the telephone, shopping for groceries, preparing meals, or going up and down stairs, because of trouble seeing?
- Are the client's clothes soiled or mismatched?
- Does the client use his or her hands to maneuver around at home?
- Are the client's prescriptive lenses current?
  (Barry, 2000, p. 378.)

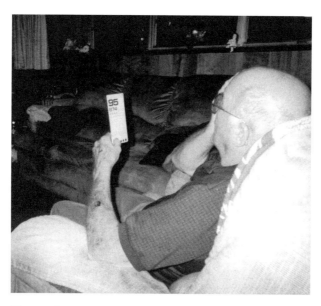

Figure 3-1 As part of the teaching/learning assessment, a vision assessment is performed in the home.

In addition to the above observations, the nurse may ask the client to read some of the educational handouts that are intended to be used in the teaching session (Figure 3-1). If the client's visual deficits have not been reported to the client's physician, then it is appropriate to do so at this time.

Hearing   The loss of hearing and/or hearing impairment alters an individual's quality of life by limiting activities such as communicating, enjoying music, listening to grandchildren playing, and enjoying the sounds of the environment such as birds singing and streams flowing. Hearing impairment can also lead to fear, boredom, apathy, depression, social isolation, and feelings of low self-esteem (Kramer et al., 2002). Hearing deficits are not an expected result of aging; however, in the United States, an estimated 60 percent of individuals who are hearing impaired are over the age of 65. Hearing loss may be the result of age-related changes or may be related to other factors such as occupation, heredity, or chronic disease. It is thought that men experience hearing loss more frequently and earlier than women because men are frequently exposed to high levels of occupational noise. The ototoxic effects of many medications can also cause hearing deficits (Miller, 2004; Saxon & Etten, 2002).

During the home visit, the nurse-educator can supplement the admission nurse's original assessment of hearing by asking the following questions:

- Does the client have difficulty following verbal instructions or does he frequently ask you to repeat or clarify what has just been said?
- Does the client have difficulty hearing your questions or reply inappropriately?
- Does the client read your lips or mouth words you are saying?
- Does the client speak in an inappropriately loud voice?
- Does the client always try to control the conversation by speaking loudly and incessantly?

- Is the client's television extremely loud?
- Does the client have a hearing aid and use it?
  (Barry, 2000, p. 378.)

Hearing loss is insidious and often goes unnoticed by both clients and families. If the loss has gone unnoticed, it is possible that a client may be eligible for hearing improvement by using a hearing aid or assistive listening device. When the nursing assessment indicates an undiagnosed hearing loss, the nurse-educator should discuss with the client the possibility of a hearing evaluation.

Motor Function   The performance of procedures that involve motor function is often required of home care clients. Assessment of motor function requires the combined evaluation of the neurological and musculoskeletal systems. Strength, balance, reaction time, speed, and flexibility are included in the assessment of motor function (Jarvis, 2004). Age-related changes in the musculoskeletal system that have the greatest impact on function are: (1) loss of muscle mass, (2) deterioration of muscle fibers with subsequent replacement by connective tissue and eventually by fat tissue, and (3) deterioration of muscle cell membranes (Miller, 2004). These changes may make it difficult for a client to handle and manipulate small objects, like an insulin syringe. Neurological changes may cause hand tremors, and cardiopulmonary changes may limit strength and endurance. During the home visit the nurse-educator can assess deficits in motor function by asking the client to perform these simple tasks:

- Touch each finger to the thumb in sequence (coordination).
- Touch the nose (coordination).
- Pick up a small object (manipulation).
- Indicate when and where they are touched (sensory).

Literacy

Low literacy in the United States is a problem of major proportions. The National Institute for Literacy (NIFL) defines **literacy** as the "ability to read, write, and speak English proficiently, to compute and solve problems, and to use technology in order to become a lifelong learner and to be effective in the family, the workplace, and the community" (NIFL, 2000, p. 1). Low health literacy, a concern of all health care professionals, is defined as "the inability to read, understand and act on health information" (Pfizer, 2003, p. 1). The National Assessment of Adult Literacy reported that as of 2003, 30 million adults (people over the age of 16), or 14 percent of the U.S. population, are below the basic literacy category (ProLiteracy Worldwide, 2005).

Many organizations in the United States such as National Institute for Literacy (NIFL), Literacy Volunteers of America (LVA), and the Pfizer Corporation have as their goal the improvement of reading levels. The list of health information that health care clients must read and understand ranges from educational handouts to instructions on medication bottles and nutritional data on food labels. Health care professionals cannot assume that their clients can read and understand the materials given them. It is well documented that low literacy is associated with poor heath; with millions of people in the United States who read at or below the fifth-grade level, the health risks are staggering (NIFL, 2000).

People's appearance, conversational skills, or years of education cannot establish their level of literacy. Many people are accomplished at compensating for low literacy. Others may falsely claim they have read and understand health–related material to prevent the embarrassment of acknowledging low literacy. The number of years people have attended school is not necessarily an indicator of reading ability. Assurance that health care clients are able to read and understand health-related materials is best achieved by preparing materials at the sixth-grade level or lower (Winslow, 2001).

Literacy Level   Health education information is available to the general public in a variety of formats from many distributors such as magazines, newspapers, TV commercials, and pharmacies. However, written information provided by health care professionals such as home care nurses remains the primary source of information for many health care clients (Winslow, 2001). The educational materials used by nurse-educators for the teaching/learning process in home care should be readily accessible to their clients and, most importantly, should be easily understood. Frequently, this is not the case. Research has indicated that health information is often written above the literacy level of health care clients, both in home care and institutionalized care (Wilson, 2000).

Determining Literacy Level   Determining the reading level of written materials is accomplished by using formulas. The first readability formula was developed over 80 years ago, and today more than 40 readability formulas exist. Measurements used to determine readability level are the number of syllables (or letters) in a word and the number of words in a sentence. Readability levels can be calculated by hand or with computer programs. One of the oldest formulas, which is done by hand, is the SMOG Readability Formula (Table 3-3). Two popular computer formulas are the Flesch Reading Ease and the Flesch-Kincaide Grade Level, both included with Microsoft Word (Bailey, 2002; Winslow, 2001).

Health care educators who are interested in calculating the readability level of their written materials may find the SMOG Readability Formula among the easiest to use. Instructions for the use of SMOG with materials with over 30 sentences are:

1. Block 10 sentences in a row near the beginning of your material. Count 10 sentences in the middle. Count 10 sentences near the end (30 sentences total).
2. Count every word with three or more syllables in each group of sentences, even if the same word appears more than once.
3. Add the total number of words counted. Use the SMOG Conversion Table I to find the grade level (Table 3-3).

Instructions for SMOG use with materials with less than 30 sentences are:

1. Count the total number of sentences in the material.
2. Count the number of words with three or more syllables.
3. Find the total number of sentences and the corresponding conversion number in SMOG Conversion Table II.
4. Multiply the total number of words with three or more syllables by the conversion number. Use this number as the word count to find the correct grade level from Table I.

Box 3-2 illustrates the use of the SMOG conversion table for calculating readability level.

Cultural Background

"As a nurse enters the home of an individual or a family, the people remain alert to see whether he or she will be responsive to their cultural beliefs, values, mannerisms, dress, language, and symbols" (Leininger, 2001, p. 222). These words, by nurse-anthropologist Dr. Madeleine

---

BOX 3-2 SAMPLE USING SMOG CONVERSION TABLE I (TABLE 3-3) FOR ASSESSING READABILITY LEVEL

Step 1: Choose three blocks of 10 sentences for a total of 30 sentences.
The role of the nurse as an educator is inherent within all nurses in all health delivery settings; however, the home care nurse as an educator is an absolute necessity. Education is the vital link between the health care provider, the home care client, and the plan of care. The need for education related to the client's condition is independent of diagnosis, socioeconomic status, or age. Shorter hospital stays, higher client acuity on discharge from health care facilities, the aging population and clients' escalating need for knowledge related to their conditions have contributed to the increased

The nurse who admits a client to a home care agency will have completed a comprehensive client physical assessment prior to the development of a personalized plan of care. The nurse-educator, who may or may not be the client's admitting nurse, will use information from the physical assessment as a foundation in developing a teaching plan. Each system of the human body undergoes physical changes with the aging process. Changes that are particularly important to assess in relation to the client's ability to learn new health information are sight, hearing, and coordination. Age-related changes and their

Home care nurses are fully participating in the technological revolution in health care. Laptops and handheld computers are used for documentation of in-home visits; telemonitors are used for assessing vital signs, blood pressure, blood glucose, heart and lung sounds, oxygen saturation, and weight; and digital cameras and digital camcorders for photo documenting such as wound status. Thus, the home care nurse, in addition to traditional health teaching, has taken on the role of teaching and monitoring the use of home care equipment by clients. Certainly, this has been done for years with equipment

Step 2: Count every word of three or more syllables.
There are 60 words with three or more syllables in the previous 30 sentences.

Step 3: Add the total number of words counted. Using Conversion Table I (Table 3-3), the sample is written at a 12th-grade level.

Leininger, succinctly state the level of scrutiny directed toward home care nurses as they interact with their clients.

The United States continues to grow in diversity. The newest peoples migrating to the United States are from Mexico and Central America, the former countries of the Soviet Union, Asia, and the war-torn countries of Eastern Europe. Many of these new residents, when needing

TABLE 3-3 SMOG Conversion Tables

SMOG CONVERSION TABLE I (FOR LONGER MATERIALS)		SMOG CONVERSION TABLE II (USE WITH MATERIAL < 30 SENTENCES)	
WORD COUNT	GRADE LEVEL	NO. SENTENCES	CONVERSION NO.
0–2	4	29	1.03
3–6	5	28	1.07
7–12	6	27	1.1
13–20	7	26	1.5
21–30	8	25	1.2
31–42	9	24	1.25
43–56	10	23	1.3
57–72	11	22	1.36
73–90	12	21	1.43
91–110	13	20	1.5
111–132	14	19	1.58
133–156	15	18	1.67
157–182	16	17	1.76
183–210	17	16	1.87
211–240	18	15	2.0
		14	2.14
		13	2.3
		12	2.5
		11	2.7
		10	3.0

Source: Adapted from McLaughlin, 1969.

health-related services, will find themselves being cared for by home care nurses. Home care nurses will, in turn, find themselves with the mission of communicating home care explanations and instructions to an audience that may be leery of their message. Acceptance and respect of cultures different from our own is absolutely necessary if the message delivered by health care providers is to be believed and followed.

Particularly challenging for health care providers and clients alike is communicating accurate and complete information to clients who have little or no understanding of the English language. Federal and state laws require that full language access to health care services be available for consumers in health care agencies receiving federal funds to pay for any health care services (Perez-Stable & Napoles-Springer, 2000). The best solution to this situation is to use a trained medical interpreter who is a "specially trained professional who has proficient knowledge and skills in a primary language or languages and who

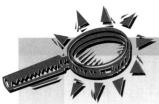

Evidenced-Based Practice Box 3-1

Culturally Tailored Health Care Teaching

Two recent research studies support the premise that culturally tailored health care teaching increases clients' ability to successfully manage their chronic illness. Wang and Chang (2005) conducted a study on Chinese-Americans with type 2 diabetes, while Lorig, Ritter, and Gonzales (2003) conducted their research on Hispanics with chronic illnesses.

Diabetes management among Chinese-Americans has been difficult because of language barriers, difficulty in lifestyle transitions, financial constraints, and incomplete acculturation. Forty Chinese-Americans participated in a community education program that included certified diabetes educators who spoke Mandarin, Cantonese, or Taiwanese; dietary education that focused on common Chinese foods; use of rice bowls, soup bowls, and Chinese cooking utensils to teach serving sizes; encouragement of exercise that included Taichi and Chi-gong; and sensitivity to Chinese holidays in establishing the teaching calendar.

The growing prevalence and severity of chronic disease among the Hispanic population has highlighted the need for health care self-management. Chronic diseases represented among participants in this research study were heart disease, lung disease, and type 2 diabetes. Teachers in the Chronic Disease Self-Management Program all spoke fluent Spanish. Because the Hispanic population values their extended families, family and friends were invited to attend classes along with the research participants. Topics discussed were similar to those taught the Chinese group except with a Hispanic focus.

Results for the Chinese group were loss of weight, reduction in blood pressure, and a decrease in the HbA1c lab results. Results for the Hispanic group were demonstrated improvement in health status, health efficacy, and fewer emergency room visits.

(Lorig, Ritter, & Gonzalez, 2003; Wang & Chan, 2005).

employs that training in medical or health-related settings to make possible communications among parties speaking different languages" (Romero, 2004, p. 2720). Although medical interpreters are the best solution, the client may not agree. Some clients may prefer that family members act as interpreters, believing that their quality of care will be better. Additionally, trained interpreters may be available in large medical centers but are rare in small facilities. The laws are well intentioned but interpreters have not been as available and useful as intended (Romero, 2004).

Culture, as it relates to clients in nursing, is not just a matter of addressing needs of people from other countries or ethnic backgrounds. Cultural groups include (1) people of one gender, (2) people of a particular age group, (3) people who are in compromised social conditions, (4) people from specific geographic areas within this country, (5) people who are clinging to their original culture, (6) people who live in ethnic communities within the United States, and (7) people immigrating to the United States. Diversity in the United States means "that nurses who work in multicultural settings will be responsible for recognizing the broad differences in beliefs and practices of various cultural groups and for developing strategies (often different from mainstream or conventional methods) for client education" (Wilson, 2000, p. 109).

Health practices in the home care setting that may influence family participation in the client's care are cognitive abilities especially if English is not spoken in the home; acceptance of medications, treatments, and therapies that may be new to the client; and reluctance to adhere to modalities that are not covered by insurance, Medicare, or Medicaid. The home care nurse-educator, by respecting and attempting to include the beliefs of the client, may find that implementing the educational plan is more successful than expected.

Teaching

The following quote aptly describes the enormous expectations placed on nurse-educators: "Clients, families, administrations, quality improvement staff members, referral sources, physicians, and Medicare surveyors expect nurses and other clinicians to be expert teachers" (Martin, 2000, p. 116). With an understanding about how people learn and after a thorough assessment of the conditions under which teaching/learning will occur, the nurse-educator is ready to begin the teaching/learning process.

Development of a Teaching/Learning Plan

Development of a teaching/learning plan is similar to the development of a nursing care plan. The steps are (1) assessing learning needs and readiness to learn, (2) identifying goals and developing learning objectives, (3) implementing the plan, and (4) evaluating the plan. Like a nursing care plan, the learning objectives will be derived from the client assessment. Home care agencies have standardized teaching/learning plans for the majority of conditions that the home care nurse will encounter. These plans serve as a framework for individualizing a teaching/learning plan.

The purpose of the teaching/learning plan, which is built around the client's needs, is to provide a framework for the health care professionals who will be conducting the teaching. The plan should include the following:

- What type of information is to be taught.
- When the information is to be taught.
- Where the teaching will take place.
- How the teaching will be done.
- Who will do the teaching.
  (Falvo, 2004, p. 88.)

Health care practitioners should not make assumptions about a client's knowledge related to the condition that has warranted home care services. A conversational approach about the condition will quickly clue the nurse to the client's level of understanding. Lack of understanding may be related to impaired cognition, or it may be that a client simply is not similar with his diagnosis. After the initial assessments, ask the client what he wants to know about his care and condition. Using the client's responses, the nurse and client can progress to setting goals. When the client and nurse agree on the goals, then the client/nurse team progresses to a teaching plan. Such an approach makes clients partners in managing their own health. Enthusiasm on the part of the nurse for the teaching/learning process enhances success (Bruccoliere, 2000; London, 2001; Sitzman, 2001; Washburn, 2000).

Assessing Learning Needs and Readiness to Learn   Being a home care client with a health-threatening condition is for most people an anxiety-producing situation. Additionally, the prospect of having to learn new information, taught by someone who is unknown to the client or the client's family, adds to an already trying situation. It is the wise nurse who recognizes that these factors enter into the teaching/learning mix. A conversation about fears, stress, and the unknown is appropriate with a client who appears to be anxious. Mild anxiety can be a motivator to learn; however, as any nursing student will agree, moderate or severe stress may be an impediment to learning (Barry, 2000; Bruccoliere, 2000).

The home care nurse having assessed the client's physical and mental abilities, cultural background, and literacy level now must assess the client's learning needs and readiness to learn. Either the nurse or the client may recognize the client's need for information. A client who asks, "How will I give myself insulin?" has identified her own need for knowledge. Although readiness to learn occurs when the prospective learner recognizes her learning needs, there are other conditions that must be favorable such as freedom from physical discomfort and anxiety, a timeframe that is comfortable for both the learner and the educator, and a feeling that now is the time to start (Falvo, 2004).

It is helpful to select a time for the teaching visit that is agreeable to both the nurse and the client. It is also helpful to begin the teaching/learning session by asking clients and families, when appropriate, where they receive their health information. Answers to this inquiry will assist the nurse in knowing where to begin. Responses will range from not knowing where to look to searching the Internet. The nurse-educator having reviewed the physical assessment may have to immediately address physical limitations. First and foremost, the client cannot be uncomfortable or in pain. When necessary, pain control must be addressed prior to continuing with the teaching session.

Identifying Goals and Developing Learning Objectives   The client who finds herself in a health-compromised condition may have to learn new information that, until now, was not necessary for her to know. For example, the client who is recently diagnosed with diabetes mellitus may have to learn about the following: (1) the disease process, (2) nutrition, (3) exercise, (4) medications, (5) glucose testing, (6) insulin administration, (7) adverse effects of medications, and (8) signs and symptoms of disease complications. This much information may take several teaching/learning sessions over a period of weeks. Each topic will necessitate a goal followed by objectives. Bastable (2003) makes clear the distinction between goals and objectives by stating:

> The goal is the final outcome of what is to be achieved. Goals are global and broad in nature. Goals are the desired outcomes of learning that are realistically achievable in weeks or months, whereas, an objective is a specific, single, one-dimensional behavior. It is short-term in nature and should be achieved at the end of one teaching session (p. 321).

Some home care clients will need help with medical/nursing language and interpretation of medical terminology. In such a case, it is wise to define all complex medical terms and to break the teaching segments into short sessions. Additionally, if the client's primary language is not English, then an interpreter may be needed. When a trained medical interpreter is not available, a family member may be available to serve as an interpreter (Bruccoliere, 2000; Sitzman, 2001).

Learning needs derive from the assessment and are established by the client and nurse. Once the learning needs have been established, goals and objectives are written in precise

---

BOX 3-3 SUMMARY OF TEACHING TIPS

- Assess vision, hearing, and motor function.
- Assess mental status and readiness to learn.
- Assess literacy level.
- Develop with the client a teaching plan.
- Establish with the client learning objectives.
- Use black letters on white or light background for written materials.
- Use size 14 font or higher.
- Avoid using all uppercase letters.
- Sit in front of the client when speaking.
- Shut off background noise.
- Speak slowly.
- Use lay terminology when possible.
- State objectives clearly and succinctly.
- Introduce the possibility of using the Internet.

---

language. For example, a home care nurse is working with a client who has been newly diagnosed with type 2 diabetes mellitus. The nurse and client agree that it is necessary for her to learn how to monitor her blood glucose. In developing learning objectives related to blood glucose testing two possible objectives are (1) the client will correctly state the steps necessary to test blood glucose levels and (2) the client will correctly test her blood glucose level. Note that the first objective only requires that the client state the steps necessary for glucose testing, whereas the second objective requires that the learner perform the glucose testing correctly. An objective includes the acceptable level of accuracy. A familiar example is in CPR classes, where the learner must pass the written test at 84 percent or better. In the example of the glucose testing, there is only one acceptable level of accuracy.

A sample teaching plan is illustrated in Figure 3-2.

Implementing the Plan   Once the learning needs have been identified and the objectives have been agreed upon, the teaching begins. Ideally, one health care professional will conduct all of the teaching sessions. When this is not possible, communication between all of the teachers is a must. Each needs to know the progress that has been made and what remains to be done. Consistency among the teachers helps ensure the effectiveness of client education.

Nurse-educators should view the teaching/learning plan as a plan that is always in progress; therefore, alterations are always a possibility. In home care, implementation of the teaching plan is almost always one-on-one, allowing for continuous assessment. Alterations in the plan or in the use of teaching materials may be necessary as new client needs are identified. Although evaluation of the plan is the last step in the process, evaluation begins at the first teaching session.

Evaluation of the Teaching/Learning Plan   The importance of evaluating the outcomes of teaching/learning has never been more crucial than in today's health care environment.

Teaching Plan for Self-monitoring Glucose Level   (25 Minutes)

Goal: The client will correctly test and document blood glucose level

Objectives	Instruction	Time	Evaluation
The client will be able to:			
Identify the monitor parts:			
• Point to the on/off button.	Demonstrate and request a return demonstration.	5 minutes	Completed
• Identify the display screen.			
• Open the battery pocket.			
• Identify the strip slot.			
• Identify a test strip.			
Prepare the monitor for use:			
• Turn the monitor on correctly.	Instruct the client that the monitor is ready for use.	5 minutes	Completed
• Observe for 3 numbers.			
• Observe a picture of a drop of blood.			
• Remove a strip from the test strip vial.			
• Replace the vial cap tightly.			
• Insert strip (window up) into the strip slot.			

Figure 3-2 *(Continues)*

Place a drop of blood on the test strip using a lancet pen:		
• Pull the cap off the lancet (pen) correctly?	Demonstrate use of lancet pen.	10 minutes	Completed
• Insert a lancet firmly in place.	Wash hands.	5 minutes	Completed
• Replace the cap.	Obtain drop of blood		
• Wash hands.	from self and place on		
• Hang arm down by side.	test strip.		
• Select finger to be pricked.			
• Place the lancet pen against the finger.			
• Press the button.			
• Place drop of blood on strip correctly.	Ask for a repeat demonstration.	5 minutes	Completed
• Wait for the reading.			
Record the glucose reading:			
• Read the result number correctly.	Ask client to identify the glucose reading and record in the log.	5 minutes	Completed
• Record the test result in log.			

Figure 3-2 Sample teaching/learning plan (*Continued*)

Evaluation measures the level of success in meeting stated goals and objectives. Positive outcomes resulting from successful teaching/learning plans include reduction in length of hospital stays, reduction in costs both for the clients and third-party payers, and improved client outcomes (Rankin & Stallings, 2001).

The one-on-one teaching/learning that occurs in home care allows for immediate evaluation of the client's learning. Whether it is recall of significant information or evaluation of a psychomotor skill, both the nurse and client can know immediately if the session was completely successful or if more work needs to be done in a particular area (Rankin & Stallings, 2001). The teaching plan in Figure 3-2 includes evaluation of glucose-testing skill.

Documentation of the Teaching/Learning Plan   Home care nurses have long known the importance of accurate, detailed documentation. In teaching the client, documentation revolves around the teaching plan. Documentation will include the client's response to the teaching/learning materials, which objectives have been met, amount of time needed for meeting each objective, and objectives that remain unmet.

Technology and Teaching

During the last ten years the technology of communication systems has experienced phenomenal growth—a growth that has altered the retrieval and management of information in health care delivery systems. The changes affect all aspects of health care.

Home care nurses are fully participating in the technological revolution in health care. Laptops and handheld computers are used for documentation of in-home visits; telemonitors are used for assessing vital signs, blood pressure, blood glucose, heart and lung sounds, oxygen saturation, and weight; and digital cameras and digital camcorders for photo documenting such as wound status (Chetney & Sauls, 2003; Demarest, & Acoraci, 2004; Durtschi, 2001; Kobb, Hilsen, & Ryan, 2003). Thus, the home care nurse, in addition to traditional health teaching, has taken on the role of teaching and monitoring the use of home care equipment by clients. Certainly, this has been done for years with equipment such as PCA pumps and glucose monitors. Now, teaching includes the use of the telemonitor, proper adjustment of the camera, proper placement of stethoscopes and blood pressure cuffs, and the use of equipment used in teleconferences.

In addition to the use of technology in the clinical aspects of client care, nurses and clients are turning to technology for educational purposes. Home care telehealth educational programs recently reported in the literature include the University of Connecticut School of Nursing Personal Education Program, which helps older adults learn about interactions associated with over-the-counter medications; the Cardiac Connection Program, managed by a home care agency in Virginia; and in Oregon, tele-home teaching provided to clients and families of clients with diabetes and hypertension (Chetney, 2003; Durtschi, 2001; Nealsey, 2003).

Advantages of tele-home care are well documented and include reduction of hospitalizations, reduction in length of in-client days, better client outcomes, and higher client satisfaction. "Success results from the technology allowing nurses to have more communication with their clients" (Kinsella 2003, p. 662). Refer to Chapter 12 for a detailed discussion of technology in home care.

The gap in computer competence among home care clients ranges from those clients who have never turned on a computer to those who access the World Wide Web for information about health-related conditions and, in some cases, access to support groups for assistance in coping with health problems. The Pew Internet & American Life Project, an arm of the Pew

Research Center, tracks all aspects of computer life among Americans. Findings of interest to home care professionals are the following:

- Eight million Americans age 65 or older use the Internet.
- This number represents an increase of 45 percent between 2000 and 2004.
- 66 percent of seniors on-line have used the Internet to seek medical information (Pew Internet and American Life Project, 2004).

The percentage of seniors who use the Internet is still considerably less than the population in general; however, as the baby boomers come of age, predictions are that the use of technology and the Internet will increase accordingly.

Summary

The partnership between the home care nurse-educator and the home care client is at the core of home care. Successful teaching/learning helps not only the client, but the client's family, nurse, and community. The improvement in quality of life is immeasurable for the client and family who understand the client's condition and treatments.

This chapter discussed the history of several prominent learning theories with emphasis on the theory of adult learning. The teaching/learning assessment addressed the mental status, physical status, literacy level, and cultural background of the client and his or her relationship to the teaching/learning process.

Goals and objectives were discussed in relation to the development of a teaching/learning plan, as was the necessity of evaluation and documentation of the plan.

The role of the home care nurse was described as a nurse, teacher, and facilitator of learning for both client and family.

References

American Foundation for the Blind. (2004). *Quick facts and figures on blindness and low vision.* Jan. 16, 2004,
   http://www.afb/info_document_view

Bailey, B. (2002). *Readability formulas. Human Factors International,* June 2002, retrieved January 19, 2004 from
   http://humanfactors.com/downloads/jun022.htm

Barry, C. B. (2000). Teaching the older client in the home: Assessment and adoption. *Home Healthcare Nurse, 18*(6), 374–386.

Bastable, S. B. (2003). *Nurse as educator: Principles of teaching and learning for nursing practice.* (2nd. ed.). Boston: Jones and Bartlett.

Battershy, D. (1987). From andragogy to gerogogy. *Journal of Educational Gerontology, 2*(1), 4–10.

Bruccoliere, T. (2000). How to make client teaching stick. *RN, 63*(2), 34–38.

Chetney, R., & Sauls, E. (2003). A picture speaks louder than words . . . but a digital camcorder tells the whole story. *Home Healthcare Nurse, 21*(10), 694–695.

Demarest, L., & Acoraci L. R. (2004). Choosing and using a digital camera in home care. *Home Healthcare Nurse, 22*(1), 61–63.

Durtschi, A. (2001). Three clients' tele-home care experiences. *Home Healthcare Nurse, 19*(1), 9–11.

Eliopoulos, C. (2001). *Gerontological nursing.* (5th ed.). Philadelphia: Lippincott.

Falvo, D. R. (2004). *Effective patient education: A guide to increased compliance.* (3rd ed.). Sudbury, MA: Jones and Bartlett.

Huitt, W., & Hummel, J. (1997). *Observational (social) learning.* Retrieved February 9, 2004 from http://chiron.valdosta.edu/whuitt/col/soccog/soclrn.html

Jarvis, C. (2004). *Physical examination & health assessment.* (4th. ed.). St. Louis: Saunders.

Joint Commission on the Accreditation of Healthcare Organizations. (2003). *Comprehensive accreditation manual of home care.* Oakbrook Terrace, IL. Joint Commission Resources Inc. PF-1.

Joint Commission on the Accreditation of Healthcare Organizations. (2004). *Comprehensive accreditation manual of home care.* Oakbrook Terrace, IL. Joint Commission Resources Inc. PC-24.

Kinsella, A. (2003). Telehealth opportunities for home care clients. *Home Healthcare Nurse, 21*(10), 661–655.

Knowles, M. S. (1980). *The modern practice of adult education: From pedagogy to andragogy.* Chicago: Follett Publishing Co.

Kobb, R., Hilsen, P., & Ryan, P. (2003). Assessing technology needs for the elderly. *Home Healthcare Nurse, 21*(10), 667–673.

Kramer, S. E., Kapteyn, T. S., Kuik, D. J., & Deeg. D. J. H. (2002). The association of hearing impairment and chronic diseases with psychosocial health status in older age. *Journal of Aging and Health, 14,* 122–137.

Leininger, M. M. (2001). Transcultural nursing in the community. In Lundy & Janes, *Community health nursing: Caring for the public's health* (pp. 218–233). Sudbury, MA: Jones & Bartlett.

London, F. (2001). Take the frustration out of client education. *Home Healthcare Nurse, 19*(3), 158–163.

Lorig, K. R., Ritter, P. L., & Gonzalez, V. M. (2003). Hispanic chronic disease self-management. *Nursing Research, 52*(6), 361–369.

Martin, K. S. (2000). The ABCs of health education and teaching guides. *Home Care Provider, 5*(4), 116–117.

McLaughlin, G. (1969). SMOG grading: A new readability formula. *Journal of Reading, 12*(8), 639–646.

Miller, C. (2004). *Nursing for wellness in older adults* (4th. ed.). Philadelphia: Lippincott Williams & Williams.

National Association for Home Care. (2001). *Basic statistics for home care.* Retrieved January 12, 2004 from http://www.nahc.org

National Institute for Literacy. (2000*). Fact sheet: Adult and family literacy.* Retrieved January 19, 2004 from

http://www.nifl.gov

Nealsey, P. J. (2003). Interactive personal technology education program. *Home Health care Nurse, 21*(10), 697–698.

Perez-Stable, E. J., & Napoles-Springer, A. (2000). Interpreters and communication in the clinical encounter. *American Journal of Medicine, 108,* 509–510.

Pew Internet & American Life Project. (2004, March 25). *Older Americans and the Internet.* Retrieved May 10, 2004, from

http://www.pewin.../reports.asp?=117&Section=ReportLevel1&Field=Level1D&ID

Pfizer Clear Health Communication. (2003). What is health?

http://www.pfizerhealthliteracy.com

ProLiteracy Worldwide. (2005). Adult literacy figures no surprise to proliteracy worldwide. Retrieved December 29, 2005 from

http://www.literacyvolunteers.org/news/index.asp?aid=136

Rankin, S. H., & Stallings. K. D. (2001). *Client education: Principles & practice.* (4th. ed.). Philadelphia: Lippincott.

Redman, B. K. (2001). *The practice of client education.* (9th. ed.). St. Louis: Mosby.

Romero, C. M. (2004). Using medical interpreters. *American Family Physician, 69*(11), 2720, 2722.

Saxon, S. V., & Etten, M. J. (2002). *Physical change & aging.* (4th. ed.). New York: Tiresias Press.

Sitzman, K. (2001). Tips for teaching older adults. *Home Healthcare Nurse, 19*(3), 141.

Smith, M. K. (2002). Malcolm Knowles, informal adult education, self-direction and andragogy. *The encyclopedia of informal education,* http://www.infed.org/thinkers/et-knowl.htm Last updated April 05, 2002. Retrieved Jan. 13, 2004.

Townsend, M. C. (2000). *Psychiatric mental health nursing: Concepts of care.* (3rd. ed.). Philadelphia: F. A. Davis.

Wang, C., & Chan, S. M. A. (2005). Culturally tailored diabetes education program for Chinese Americans. *Nursing Research, 54*(5), 347–353.

Washburn, P. V. (2000). How to improve client education. *Hospital Topics, 78*(4), 5–8.

Wilson, F. L. (2000). Are client information materials too difficult to read? *Home Healthcare Nurse, 18*(2), 107–115.

Winslow, E. H. (2001). Client education materials: Can clients read them, or are they ending up in the trash? *American Journal of Nursing, 101*(10), 33–38.

Chapter 4

Infection Control

Kathleen Hoehn, RN, BSN

Key Terms

Community-Acquired
Methicillin-resistant
Staphylococcus aureus

Contact Precautions

Direct Observation
Therapy

Hand Hygiene

Methicillin-resistant
Staphylococcus aureus
(MRSA)

Personal Protective
Equipment

Pulmonary Tuberculosis

Standard Precautions

T he complexity of infection control in the home care setting can be challenging both for the health care worker and the client, for several reasons. Drug-resistant bacteria have moved their residence from hospitals to client homes. The client's home may have evolved into a mini-hospital complete with hospital bed, walker, bedside commode, IV pole, pump, bag, and tubing. Home care clients, in general, have some knowledge about infections. However, they do not always follow basic principles. It is important to provide basic infection-control education to clients and their caregivers during home care services.

This chapter is written to promote the safety of home care employees and home care clients. Information contained here is intended to educate all involved with the provision of home health services about infection control in the home, with a goal of preventing the spread of infection and achieving optimum client outcomes. Included in this chapter is information about the "chain of infection," infectious organisms in the home, and tools for infection control in home care.

Chain of Infection

The chain of infection (Figure 4-1) is a graphic representation of events in an infectious process that may lead to the development of active infection.

In addition to an infectious agent and susceptible host, there must be a reservoir or source, a portal of exit from the source, a mode of transmission, and a portal of entry into the host. In between each step are actions by health care personnel that can be taken to break the chain of infection. These actions can help control the interaction between the agent and the host.

For example, cleaning of equipment used in the home care visit will break the chain of infection by eliminating the *infectious agent*. Another example, the covering of mouth and nose when coughing or sneezing, will eliminate the *portal of exit* from the source. Proper hand hygiene will interrupt the *mode of transmission* of an infectious agent. The use of

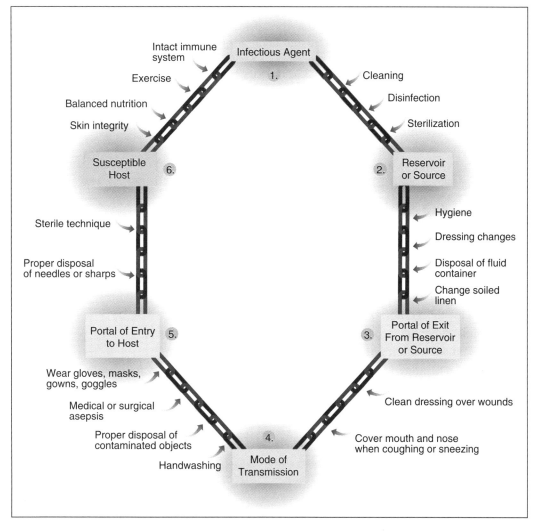

Figure 4-1 Chain of infection *(Source: DeLaune & Ladner, 2006.)*

sterile technique when performing dressing changes will prevent a *portal of entry* to the host. And finally, maintenance of skin integrity will protect a *susceptible host*.

Infection-Control Program

The goal of an Infection-Control Program is to reduce the risk of transmission of infection among clients and employees. Home care agencies incorporate control strategies into their plan for infection control. Examples of these strategies include:

- Targeted surveillance to identify and record infections associated with agencies, employees, and clients.
- Prevention and control of infection through employee health and safety initiatives, provision of **personal protective equipment (PPE)** (gowns, gloves, and masks used as barriers to infection), vaccinations, and tuberculosis (TB) screening.

PPE is meant to be used to prevent the spread of infection as transmitted by home care employees to other clients who may be immunocompromised and predisposed to infection.

Focused or Targeted Infection Surveillance

Home care agencies select focused infection surveillance of service lines, high-risk or high-volume procedures, or special programs as appropriate to their agency population. Focused surveillance enables the home care agency to:

- Monitor and treat client and employee infections.
- Identify commonalities in organisms and employees.
- Identify agency-associated infections.
- Aggregate data, including clusters of employee/client infections.
- Provide appropriate education to staff and clients.

Employee Health

Home care agencies promote the health of all employees and clients of a home care agency (including nurses, therapists, home health aides, social workers, and office workers) through:

- Timely referral of information regarding infections.
- Annual tuberculosis testing.
- Hepatitis B immunization (voluntary).
- National Institute for Occupational Safety and Health (NIOSH) approved masks for the care of TB infected clients.
- Safety needles.
- PPE such as gowns, gloves, and masks.
- Promotion and provision of flu vaccinations.
- Occupational exposure/injury plan and procedure, including provision of antiviral medication for high-risk exposures.
- Work restrictions related to illness.
- Employee education at the time of orientation and annually about blood-borne pathogens, drug-resistant organisms, evolving communicable diseases, and standard precautions education.

Clients are discharged home from acute care hospitals earlier in their hospital stay and with more unresolved medical conditions than in prior years. Rehabilitation hospitals and nursing facilities also discharge their clients to the care of a home health agency when needed. Prior to the client's discharge, the discharging facility should communicate information regarding the client's case including infectious diagnoses, thus allowing the home care agency the opportunity to initiate appropriate protective protocols.

Several general principles of infection control that apply to home care are:

- The home care employee should be careful to use the PPE, safety needles, and TB masks to fully protect themselves and their clients from exposures.
- The home care employee should report all occupational exposures including exposures to blood-borne and respiratory infections to agency management immediately after the incident.
- Surgical masks should be worn in any client's home where droplet infection is evident.
- Appropriate use of PPE for home care employees includes both the client's diagnosis and the condition of the home.
- Home care employees should not work with evidence of personal contagious illness such as fever, productive cough, and rashes.
- Home care employees should observe principles of good personal hygiene to minimize the transmission of disease. The following are guidelines:
  - Rings should be kept at a minimum.
  - Sleeves should be short or capable of being pushed up to a level that facilitates washing of the wrist during hand hygiene.
  - Hair should be worn in a style that will prevent contamination of clients, supplies, or equipment when leaning forward.
  - A clean lab jacket should be worn during visits.
  - Hands and fingers should be kept away from the face, nose, and mouth.
  - Areas of contact with contaminated articles must be washed with soap and water.
  - Makeup, lip balm, or contact lens must not be applied in the client area.

Infectious Organisms in Home Care

The home care employee making visits to home care clients may be the first to identify symptoms of a health threat to the client/community. The description, prevention, and treatment of several of the more common infectious and communicable diseases found in the home are now discussed. Table 4-1 illustrates the incidence, home care treatments, availability of vaccines, and preventable measures other than vaccination that are utilized in controlling these communicable conditions.

Pulmonary Tuberculosis

Pulmonary tuberculosis (TB) is an infectious disease caused by *Mycobacterium tuberculosis*. This infection is spread through airborne particles when persons with pulmonary TB sneeze, cough, speak, or sing. A person exposed to an individual with infectious TB should be given a tuberculin skin test. The Mantoux intradermal tuberculin skin test is the preferred method of skin testing. The site is examined 48 to 72 hours later for induration (a palpable,

TABLE 4-1 Incidence, Home Care Treatment, Availability of Vaccines and Preventable Measures other than Vaccines of Common Communicable Diseases Found in the Home

ORGANISM	INCIDENCE IN UNITED STATES	HOME CARE TREATMENT	PREVENTION BY VACCINE	PREVENTION OTHER THAN VACCINE
Pulmonary Tuberculosis	14,000 cases annually.	Compliance with medication regime. Infected client should wear an NIOSH respiratory protective device during caregiving activities. Discontinue precautions only when client on effective therapy is improving clinically and has three consecutive sputum smears negative for acid-fast bacillus collected on separate days.	No vaccine.	Focus on treating persons with inactive TB infections with anti-TB medications for 6–12 months.
Pertussis	5000–7000 cases/year.	Antimicrobial therapy. Stay at home unit 5–7 days of treatment with antibiotic. Bed rest. Small frequent feedings and push fluids.	Vaccine at 2, 4, 6 and 15–18 mos; 4–6 yrs and 11–12 yrs.	Prevent face-to-face contamination with a contagious individual. Exposed individuals should receive antimicrobial prophylaxis.
Influenza	• 2,000,000 hospitalized from flu complications • 36,000 die from flu. 5%–20% of population	Influenza antiviral medications.	Vaccine yearly for: residents of long term care facilities people 2–64 years with chronic health problems. Vaccine yearly > 50. Pregnant women. Health care personnel who provide direct patient care.	Get vaccinated. Good Health Habits = Avoid close contact, stay home when ill, wash hands, avoid touching eyes, nose or mouth. Health care workers follow routine barrier precautions.

TABLE 4-1 (Continues)				
ORGANISM	**INCIDENCE IN UNITED STATES**	**HOME CARE TREATMENT**	**PREVENTION BY VACCINE**	**PREVENTION OTHER THAN VACCINE**
HIV	40,000 persons become infected yearly.	Educate the caregiver on: the disease physical care, emotional support, guarding against infections, caregiver protection, and final arrangements.	Research & development ongoing in US.	Safe sex practices. IV drug users never share needles. Screening of voluntary blood donors. Health care workers use standard precautions.
Hepatitis B	73,000 in 2003 down from 260,000 per year in the 1980s. 1.25 million chronically infected in US. 5000 die from complications of hepatitis B.	Family must be educated in prevention measures such as not sharing eating utensils or bath towels. Avoid alcohol and acetaminophen. Avoid close personal contact including sexual. Adequate rest with progressive ambulation and exercise.	Vaccine Birth, 2 mos, 12–15 mos; adults 3 does (0, 1–2, 4–6 mos). Vaccination of risk groups at all ages and health care workers in direct contact with patients.	Get vaccinated. Blood test for hepatitis B if pregnant. No IV durgs. Never share needles. If multiple sex partners, use latex condoms correctly. Health care workers follow routine barrier precautions.
Hepatitis C	30,000 in 2003 down from 240,000 per year in the 1980s. 2.7 million Americans currently infected.	Same as with Hepatitis B.	No vaccine.	No IV drugs. Never share needles. If multiple sex partners use latex condoms correctly. Don't share personal items that may have blood on them (razors, toothbrushes). Health care personnel always follow routine barrier precautions.

TABLE 4-1 (Continued)

ORGANISM	INCIDENCE IN UNITED STATES	HOME CARE TREATMENT	PREVENTION BY VACCINE	PREVENTION OTHER THAN VACCINE
Severe Acute Respiratory Syndrome (SARS)	Total of 8,098 people world wide in 2003, 774 died. In US only eight reported cases.	During time of fever and 10 days after resolution of fever client should: wear a NIOSH approved respiratory device during caregiving activities or if not possible a surgical mask, have private bed and bath, have a single caregiver, have limited persons living in household and limited visitors. Caregiver should: use gloves and gown during caregiving activities and use face protection within 3 feet of the client.	No vaccine.	Travelers to China should: avoid visiting live food markets or wildlife from these markets. In case of a reemergence of SARS, travelers to areas reporting SARS should avoid settings where transmission is likely to occur such as health care facilities.
MRSA & CA-MRSA	About 25–30% of the US population in colonized with *staphylococcus aureus* approximately 1% is colonized with MRSA.	Strict hand washing. Caregiver to wear gloves during wound care. Gown, mask/eye protection when splashes are likely. Keep wounds and lesions covered with clean, dry bandages. No sharing of personal items.	No vaccine.	Practice good hygiene: keep hands clean, keep cuts and abrasion clean and covered with clean bandage until healed, Avoid contact with other people's wounds or bandages, avoid sharing personal items.

TABLE 4-1

ORGANISM	INCIDENCE IN UNITED STATES	HOME CARE TREATMENT	PREVENTION BY VACCINE	PREVENTION OTHER THAN VACCINE
Vancomycin Resistant *Enterococcus*	Rare, usually infected clients have several underlying health conditions or previous infections with MSRA.	Same as for MRSA.	No vaccine.	Same as for MRSA.
Pediculosis [(lice) (head and body)]	Head lice common but incident information unreliable. Body lice common among the homeless and people who do not have access to bathing and clean clothes. Information on incidence unreliable.	Use prescribed or OTC medications as directed.	No vaccine.	Persons infected with head lice are usually children. Avoid head to head contact when playing and avoid use of head attire between children. Boyd lice: avoid crowded conditions, bath frequently and change clothes as necessary.
Scabies	Common and world wide. Information on incidence is unreliable.	Treatment with prescribed skin lotion. Avoid close contact with other persons. All persons in household may be prescribed treatment.	No vaccine.	Good general hygiene. Avoid sharing clothes and bedding.

(DeLaune & Ladner, 2006)

raised, hardened area). If the skin test is positive or if symptoms are suggestive of TB (fever, chills, loss of appetite, weight loss, night sweats, productive cough), a chest x-ray is performed to detect TB lesions.

TB is often curable if it is diagnosed early and if effective treatment is instituted without delay. Clients with active TB are usually treated with a four-drug regimen. Preventive therapy with isoniazid (INH) can be offered to certain high-risk groups with positive tuberculin reactions based on age and size (in mm) of induration. Health care workers with occupational exposure to TB should be considered for preventive therapy if they have a positive tuberculin reaction.

Home care clients are sometimes placed on **direct observation therapy (DOT),** which is a program to ensure client compliance with TB medication regimens. DOT is usually administered through the county health department, and involves nurses who visit the client with a frequency varying from daily to several times a week to administer TB medications. DOT can prevent the evolution of drug-resistant TB by assuring that the home care client takes all the medications ordered at the prescribed frequency and for the prescribed amount of time (CDC, 2005a).

Pertussis

Pertussis is a highly communicable disease caused by the infectious agent *Bordetella pertussis,* and is usually manifested in children. Signs and symptoms include paroxysmal spasms of severe coughing, whooping, and post-tussive vomiting. In the United States, the incidence of pertussis has increased steadily since the 1980's. The incidence in 2002 was 8,296 reported cases (CDC, 2005b).

Pertussis is usually preventable via a childhood vaccine. Transmission occurs through direct contact with respiratory discharges. At risk are children too young to be fully vaccinated and those who have not completed their vaccination series. Major complications such as pneumonia, encephalopathy, seizures, and even death are most common among infants and young children. Adolescents and adults become susceptible when immunity wanes; however, the disease is often milder in adults than in infants and children (CDC, 2005b; Maine, 2004).

Influenza and Avian Influenza

Influenza (the "flu") is a contagious respiratory illness caused by influenza viruses. Infection with influenza viruses can result in mild to severe and life-threatening complications, especially in young children, the elderly, and people who are immune compromised. According to the Centers for Disease Control and Prevention (CDC), an average of 200,000 people are hospitalized for flu-related complications and 36,000 Americans die each year from complications of the flu (CDC, 2005c). Symptoms of the flu include high fever, headache, extreme tiredness, muscle aches, sore throat, dry cough, and a runny or stuffy nose. Influenza viruses are spread from person to person in respiratory droplets when someone coughs or sneezes. Strategies to stay healthy include hand-washing; avoiding touching the nose, eyes, or mouth; covering mouth and nose with a tissue when coughing or sneezing; avoiding close contact with people who are sick; and staying home when you are sick. Vaccinations that may prevent or shorten the course of the illness are offered each year in the fall. Once infected, there are antiviral drugs that can reduce the symptoms accompanying the flu.

Avian influenza, although not seen in the United States, is discussed here because of the worldwide interest it has generated. It is an emerging, evolving infectious disease. This infectious disease is a disease of birds caused by type A strains of the influenza virus. The World Health Organization (WHO) had documented 252 cases with 148 deaths, all in Asia and the

Middle East, as of October 2005. Close contact with live infected poultry is the cause of illness. It is possible that an avian influenza virus could change so that it could infect more humans and could spread easily from person to person. Control measures include quarantine of infected farms and destruction of infected or potentially exposed flocks (WHO, 2004; WHO, 2005).

HIV/AIDS and Hepatitis

HIV and hepatitis are two illnesses that place clients and health care workers at risk. According to the CDC, the estimated number of diagnosed cases of AIDS through 2003 in the United States was 929,985 (CDC, 2005d).

Hepatitis B is a serious blood-borne disease caused by the hepatitis B virus (HBV) that attacks the liver. There are about 73,000 hepatitis infections per year. More importantly and of more impact to home care employees is the fact that the CDC estimates that 1.25 million Americans are chronically infected with hepatitis B. The hepatitis B vaccine has been available since 1982 (CDC, 2005e).

Hepatitis C is a liver disease caused by the hepatitis C virus (HCV), which is found in the blood of persons who have the disease. Hepatitis C is spread by contact with the blood of an infected person, placing health care and emergency medical personnel at risk to exposure to the hepatitis virus. There is no vaccine to prevent hepatitis C (CDC, 2005f).

It is important for home care employees to protect themselves from these viruses by being vaccinated, following routine barrier precautions, and safe needle and sharps handling.

Severe Acute Respiratory Syndrome (SARS)

Severe acute respiratory syndrome (SARS) is a viral respiratory illness, which was first reported in Asia in February 2003. SARS is an evolving threat to the community. Initial signs and symptoms of SARS are high fever (>100.4°F), headache, an overall feeling of discomfort, body aches, and mild respiratory symptoms. Most clients develop pneumonia. Deaths have been reported. Close person-to-person contact via respiratory droplets spreads SARS when an infected person coughs or sneezes (CDC, 2004a).

Health care personnel may come into direct contact with the respiratory secretions of a client with SARS. Home care personnel may help with rapid recognition and response to a SAR-infected client. The client with signs and symptoms of SARS should be asked about recent travel outside the United States, particularly to Asia and Europe. The client's physician should be contacted regarding the symptomatic client with a travel history. The physician will then notify the local health department. Early diagnosis is important to the recovery of the client and also breaks the chain of infection through identification and quarantine of clients and contacts.

Multidrug-Resistant Organisms

Resistance of disease-producing organisms to antibiotic therapy has become one of the world's most serious public health threats. A major factor associated with the problem is the misuse of antibiotics (CDC, 2004b). Several of the most resistant organisms are now discussed.

Methicillin-resistant *Staphylococcus aureus* (MRSA)   MRSA is a strain of *Staphylococcus aureus* that is resistant to special beta-lactam drugs used to treat these organisms. Healthy people can carry the MRSA organisms on their skin and in their noses. Among the infections that MRSA is known to cause are wound infections, urinary tract infections, and pneumonia. Some people are carriers, and others can become infected through infections such as boils, wound infections, and pressure ulcers. MRSA can also be spread through indirect contact by touching objects in the environment. Environmental examples are towels, sheets, wound dressings, clothes, workout areas, and sports equipment contaminated by the infected skin/body fluids of a person with MRSA (CDC, 2005h; CDC, 2003). Vancomycin intravenously is the drug of choice for treatment.

Once *infected* (the organism is present and is causing illness) or *colonized* (the organism is present in or on the body but is not causing illness), clients may harbor MRSA for months or years.

Characteristics of *infection* are:

- Presence of microorganisms.
- Evidence of damage to host such as elevated temperature, purulent sputum, or purulent drainage from sites such as surgical wounds or decubitus ulcers.

Characteristics of *colonization* are:

- Presence of microorganisms.
- No apparent damage to host and no signs or symptoms of infection (such as purulent drainage).
- Microorganisms can be transmitted via the hands of colonized persons to immunosuppressed clients, who then become infected and symptomatic. To prevent this spread, hand hygiene is imperative (CDC, 2005i) Hand hygiene will be discussed later in this chapter.

Community-Acquired Methicillin-resistant *Staphylococcus aureus*   It is of interest to home care practitioners that the CDC documents certain strains of MRSA that were once largely confined to hospitals and long-term care facilities but are now emerging in the community. These strains have been named **community-acquired Methicillin-resistant *Staphylococcus aureus*, or CA-MRSA**. Community prevalence rates are rising. Recent reports document colonization and transmission in populations lacking risk factors. The origins of CA-MRSA are under investigation. Deaths of children with community-acquired MRSA strains have been reported. These children lacked risk factors for MRSA infection (CDC, 2005h).

The CDC estimates that approximately 25 to 30 percent of the population carries MRSA. There are high rates of carriage found in injection drug users, insulin-dependent diabetics, clients with dermatologic conditions and long-term indwelling intravascular catheters, and health care workers (CDC, 2005h).

Vancomycin-Resistant *Enterococcus*   Vancomycin-resistant *Enterococcus* (VRE), along with MRSA, is a commonly encountered multidrug-resistant organism that is commonly resistant to all beta-lactam antibiotics as well as aminoglycosides. VRE is usually transmitted by the unwashed hands of personnel or through contact with contaminated objects such as stethoscopes or equipment shared between clients. Infections with VRE are found in internal organs such as the bladder and bowels (CDC, 2004b).

There are two evolving classifications of *Staphylococcus* bacteria. They are Staph bacteria, which are classified as vancomycin-intermediate *Staphylococcus aureus* (VISA) and vancomycin-resistant *Staphylococcus aureus* (VRSA). Classification of VISA/VRSA is based on laboratory tests, which show how much of an antimicrobial agent is needed to inhibit the growth of the organism in a test tube. VISA and VRSA, though rare in the United States, are emerging infections. These organisms have developed a resistance to vancomycin (CDC, 2003).

The following conditions increase the risk of acquiring multidrug-resistant organisms:

- Severe illness.
- Previous exposure to antimicrobial agents.
- Underlying diseases or conditions, particularly
  - Chronic renal disease.
  - Insulin-dependent diabetes mellitus.
  - Peripheral vascular disease.
  - Dermatitis or skin lesions.
  - Conditions that weaken the immune system.
- Invasive procedures, such as
  - Dialysis.
  - Urinary catheterization.
  - Presence of invasive devices.
- Repeated contact with the health care system.
- Previous colonization by a multidrug-resistant organism.
- Advanced age.
  (CDC, 2005h.)

It is appropriate to utilize contact precautions to prevent the spread of infection of these multidrug-resistant organisms.

Pediculosis and Scabies

Pediculosis is a body, head, or pubic skin infestation by lice. The insect is visible, about 2 to 3 mm long with six legs. Areas affected are the head, neck, ears, shoulders, waist, genital region, axillae, and areas of clothing contact.

Scabies is a skin infestation by mites. Symptoms include "burrow-like" pruritic lesions on hands, webs of fingers, wrists, elbows, knees, armpits, buttocks, and waist. In immunocompromised clients, the lesions may be more widespread and may be mistaken for eczema.

For both pediculosis and scabies, home care employees should protect themselves from the risk of coming in close contact with a client suspected of having the disease. The health care provider orders a pediculicide lotion or shampoo. The family is instructed that bedding should be washed in hot water. Contact precautions are used for 24 hours or until adequate treatment has been initiated (CDC, 2005j; CDC, 2005k).

Tools for Infection Control in Home Care

Home care RNs, LPNs, therapists, home care aides, and social workers use specific tools and procedures that have been developed to prevent the spread of infection in home care. The following section describes the use of protective tools and the procedures for their use.

A review of medical and surgical asepsis is appropriate here. Medical asepsis, also called clean technique, includes any procedures used to reduce or prevent the spread of microorganisms. Hand hygiene, using gloves, and cleaning the environment are examples of clean technique. In medical asepsis, an object that is suspected of harboring organisms is considered unclean or contaminated. Surgical asepsis or sterile technique requires procedures used to eliminate all microorganisms. In sterile technique an area or object is considered contaminated if touched or exposed to an object that is not sterile.

Hand Hygiene

Hand hygiene is the process of cleaning a health care workers' hands with soap and water or alcohol gel at prescribed times. It is the single most important tool that can be used to stop the spread of infection. The home care employee should do hand hygiene:

- For a *minimum of 15 seconds.*
- Prior to and after performing each client procedure.
- After wearing gloves.
- After using the restroom.
- Prior to entry or reentry into the home care bag if client contact or a client procedure has been initiated.
- In between treatment of wounds to prevent cross-contamination.
- Prior to contact with food.

In October 2002, the CDC issued hand hygiene guidelines in *Guideline for Hand Hygiene in Health-Care Settings.* The CDC released these guidelines to improve adherence to hand hygiene in health care settings (hand-washing or use of alcohol-based hand rubs). Hand hygiene has been shown to terminate outbreaks in health care facilities, to reduce transmission of antimicrobial-resistant organisms such as methicillin-resistant *Staphylococcus aureus,* and to reduce overall infection (CDC, 2002a, 2002b).

In addition to traditional hand-washing with soap and water, the CDC is recommending the use of alcohol-based handrubs by health care personnel for client care because they address some of the obstacles that health care professionals face when taking care of clients. The advantages of alcohol-based handrubs are that they:

- Significantly reduce the number of microorganisms on the skin.
- Are fast acting and take less time to use than traditional hand-washing.
- Cause less skin irritation.

When using an alcohol-based handrub, apply the product to the palm of one hand and rub the hands together, covering all surfaces of the hands and fingernails, until the hands are dry. Note that the volume needed to reduce the number of bacteria on the hands varies by product.

The CDC emphasized that the use of gloves does not eliminate the need for hand hygiene. Likewise, the use of hand hygiene does not eliminate the need for gloves. Gloves reduce hand contamination by 70 to 80 percent, prevent cross-contamination, and protect clients and health care personnel from infection. Handrubs should be used before and after each client, just as gloves should be changed before and after each client or procedure. Additionally, the CDC guidelines state that health care personnel should avoid wearing artificial nails and keep natural nails less than one quarter of an inch long if they care for clients at high risk of acquiring infections (CDC, 2002a, 2002b).

Gloves

Gloves are an important infection-control tool. However, *gloves are not a substitute for hand hygiene.* Perform hand hygiene after *removing* gloves, because gloves could have very small holes unseen by the naked eye, or hand contamination could occur during the glove removal process. The employee could then transfer contamination or bacteria to the client's wound or skin or even to the employee's face, or to lunch items.

Transmission-Based Precautions

Categories for isolation procedures based on their mode of transmission were introduced by the CDC in 1983. In the late 1980s, in response to the risk of transmission of HIV/AIDS and other blood-borne pathogens, universal precautions were introduced. Universal precautions are now known as **standard precautions.** Standard precautions direct the home health employee to treat all human blood and body fluids as if they are infected with pathogens. This precaution includes the appropriate use of gowns, gloves, eyewear, and masks for protection from exposure to blood and body fluids. Every home care employee should utilize standard precautions for every client (Rhinehart & McGoldrick, 2006). In 1997, the CDC categorized transmission-based isolation precautions into five groups. They are contact, droplet, airborne, National Institute for Occupational Safety and Health (NIOSH) mask required, and immuno-compromised precautions.

General Precautionary Guidelines   General precautionary guidelines for transmission-based precautions are:

- Observe standard precautions always.
- Leave home care bags and laptops outside the home (car, office).
- Store PPE outside the client treatment area.
- Obtain and document physician orders for precautions.
- List isolation supplies in physician's orders.
- Notify all team members of the precautions.
- Notify paramedics, emergency room staff, and facility staff upon any client transfer.
- Chart the precautions used during your visit.

Contact Precautions   **Contact precautions** are used to interrupt person-to-person transmission of organisms that are transmitted by direct or indirect contact with the skin. Such contact occurs during caregiving activities (Rhinehart & McGoldrick, 2006). Contact precautions are built on the concept of standard precautions but add additional protection for the home care employee. Contact precautions are the most commonly used transmission-based precautions in home care.

These precautions were identified in direct response to infections caused by drug-resistant organisms such as methicillin-resistant *Staphylococcus aureus* (MRSA) and vancomycin-resistant *Enterococcus* (VRE) and the ability of these organisms to live on hands, hard surfaces, and objects in the environment for extended periods of time. The CDC recommends contact precautions in addition to standard precautions when the health care entity or regulations deem multidrug-resistant microorganisms to be of special clinical or epidemiologic significance (Rhinehart & McGoldrick, 2006).

Specifically, home care workers should focus on prevention of cross-transmission via the home care bag and equipment which is carried to and from the home by the health care professional. Alternatively, the home care bag may be left in the vehicle and only the disposable items used for the client carried into the home. Reusable equipment may be cleaned either in the client's home or bagged prior to returning to the clinician's vehicle or facility for disinfection. Home care workers may also transport organisms on their clothing. Personal protective equipment (PPE) (gowns, gloves, and/or masks) act as barriers to the transport of infectious organisms. Hand hygiene should be performed before leaving the home. To properly comply with contact precautions, home care employees should:

- Perform hand hygiene and put on PPE (gowns, gloves, and/or masks) *prior* to client or environmental contact.
- Store PPE either outside the room that the client predominately uses or, if this is not possible, store PPE away from the client's normal route through the residence, thereby protecting the PPE from contamination.
- Cover the bag or box where the PPE is stored.
- Avoid using the bathroom as a storage area for PPE due to dampness.

Often, the client's family members ask whether they need to wear the personal protective equipment left in the home by the home care agency as they care for their family member. Family members remain in the home with usually one ill person. Thus, the PPE, particularly the isolation gowns, are meant to be used by the home care employees and not the care-givers/family of the client. At the home care staff's direction, the family may use boxes of gloves left in the home. The caregiver may want to protect personal clothing by using a designated piece of clothing when providing care to the client. Education of the client and family will be discussed later in this chapter.

Family members of the client in contact precautions often ask questions about allowing the infected person to hold or touch individuals at risk for infection such as infant family members. Each case should be treated individually. It is not advisable to expose newborns or infants to the infected person; however, restrictions like this can be unacceptable to the family/client. Good judgment and careful hand hygiene by the client and family should be employed in this circumstance. Additional precautions that can be taken include wiping the infant or child's hands and mouth following contact with the infected person. Examples of organisms that require use of contact precautions are MRSA, VRE, scabies, lice, and multidrug-resistant gram-negative organisms.

Guidelines for contact precautions are:

- Use strict hand hygiene with alcohol gel following environmental or client contact using hand hygiene guidelines.
- Apply gown and gloves prior to any environmental or client contact.
- Use a mask when a client has RSV or when a splash to the face is likely to occur.
- Use eye protection when a splash to the face is likely to occur.
- Use disposable or single-use client items such as blood pressure equipment and thermometers, and leave these in the home.

Guidelines for canceling contact precautions are that canceling should be done no sooner than 48 hours after discontinuation of all appropriate antibiotics (an antibiotic reported as "intermediate or susceptible"), and then a culture of the nares for MRSA and/or the stool for VRE or multidrug-resistant gram-negative bacilli should be obtained. If that culture is negative for an epidemiologically significant organism, contact precautions may be discontinued.

Droplet Precautions   Droplet precautions, used in addition to standard precautions, are used for clients known or suspected of being infected with microorganisms transmitted by large respiratory droplets. These droplets fall out of the air and usually land within three feet of the client (Rhinehart & McGoldrick, 2006). Conditions that require the use of droplet precautions include pertussis, influenza, and meningitis. Guidelines for droplet precautions are:

- Strict hand hygiene.
- Surgical mask within three feet of the client.
- Gloves with blood/body fluid contact.
- Gown when soiling of clothes is likely to occur.
- Eye protection when splash is likely to occur.

Cancellation of droplet precautions is dependent on the disease and requires consultation with the infection-control nurse.

Airborne Precautions   Airborne precautions are used when a client is infected with an agent that can remain suspended in the air. The client, if in a hospital, would be placed in a negative-pressure room. In home care, modifications must be made. Examples of conditions that require the use of airborne precautions are chickenpox, varicella, measles, disseminated zoster, active pulmonary or laryngeal TB, and SARS. Guidelines for airborne precautions are:

- Use hand hygiene-standard.
- Don surgical mask for non-immune staff.
- Don gloves if contact with respiratory secretions or blood/fluid contact is anticipated.
- Use gown when soiling of clothes is likely to occur.
- Wear eye protection when a splash to the face is likely to occur.

Cancellation of precautions is appropriate when all chickenpox lesions are crusted and at the duration of zoster and measles. Cancellation of airborne precautions for TB clients may be initiated when the client is improving clinically and has three consecutive negative-sputum smears for acid-base bacilli collected on different days. Clients who are on airborne precautions for SARS may be removed from isolation after resolution of fever, provided respiratory symptoms are absent or improving (Rhinehart & McGoldrick, 2006).

Airborne NIOSH-Approved Respirator/Mask   The NIOSH-mask offers a higher level of respiratory protection than surgical or isolation masks. It is recommended for use by home care staff when the client is infected with an airborne infection. Examples of conditions that require an approved NIOSH respirator are pulmonary TB, laryngeal TB, an aerosolizing wound, SARS, and a situation where TB is being ruled out. Guidelines are:

- Use a NIOSH-approved respirator (N95, HEPA, PAPR).
- Wear a mask that has been individually fit tested.
- Perform hand hygiene-standard.
- Don gloves with blood/body fluid contact.
- Wear gown when soiling of clothes is likely to occur.
- Wear eye protection when a splash to the face is likely to occur.

To cancel precautions, a physician's order must be obtained for cultures. The requirement is three negative sputum cultures on three consecutive days, compliance with medications, and improvement in the client's condition.

Immunocompromised Precautions   This category of protection, also called protected environment, was developed to be used in the direct care of bone-marrow transfer and other severely immunosuppressed clients, and is seldom used in home care. Precautions are based on the physician's diagnosis and orders for immunocompromised clients. Guidelines for these precautions are:

- Use strict hand hygiene with antimicrobial soap before and after client or environmental contact even if gloves are used.
- Wear surgical mask to enter room if you have a cold or other respiratory infection.
- Don gloves with blood/body fluid contact.
- Don gown when soiling of clothes is likely to occur.
- Wear eye protection when a splash to the face is likely to occur.

Cancellation of precautions requires a physician's order.

Home Care Bag Technique

Home care employees use bag technique to maximize the efficient use of the home care bag and to assure adherence to the principles of asepsis. The following procedure is intended for use as a guideline. Staff judgment in individual settings and with individual clients will dictate appropriate use. See Procedure 4-1 for a home care bag technique.

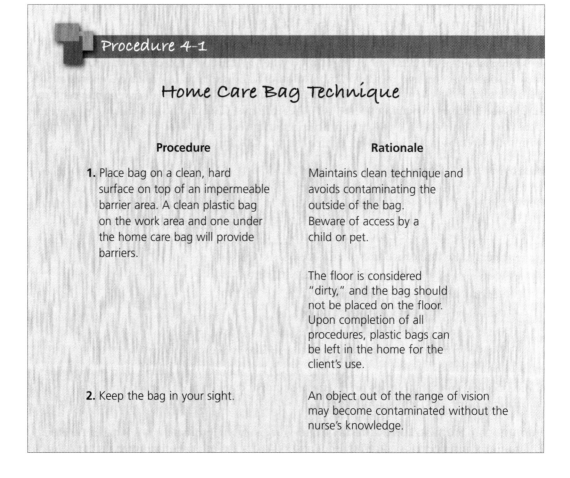

Procedure 4-1

Home Care Bag Technique

Procedure	Rationale
1. Place bag on a clean, hard surface on top of an impermeable barrier area. A clean plastic bag on the work area and one under the home care bag will provide barriers.	Maintains clean technique and avoids contaminating the outside of the bag. Beware of access by a child or pet. The floor is considered "dirty," and the bag should not be placed on the floor. Upon completion of all procedures, plastic bags can be left in the home for the client's use.
2. Keep the bag in your sight.	An object out of the range of vision may become contaminated without the nurse's knowledge.

Procedure 4-1 continued

Procedure	Rationale
3. Perform hand hygiene. Use alcohol gel or soap and towels provided by the agency.	Removes bacteria from skin surfaces and reduces transmission of organisms.
4. After hand hygiene, the home care bag may be entered.	All items in the nursing bag are considered clean; therefore, principles of medical asepsis must be followed.
5. Perform visit. Discard dirty equipment into the plastic bag. Syringes and/or sharps are disposed of in impervious containers.	Reduces transmission of organisms. Prevents sharps from puncturing sides of containers.
6. Teach the family proper disposal of dirty supplies and equipment as appropriate.	Protects family from exposure and reduces transmission of organisms.
7. Clean dirty equipment that is to be replaced in the bag and wash hands before putting equipment back in the bag.	The bag should not be taken into particularly dirty living conditions, or where a client has a communicable disease. When not in use, the bag should be stored in a clean area of the vehicle, preferably the trunk. Care should be taken to avoid extreme heat or cold.

Contents of the home care bag should be maintained in as clean a condition as possible. Home care employees need to carry supplies in their home care bags for use during client care. Several guidelines for use of the bag are:

- Home care bags usually have zippered sections and a pocket or pockets on the sides, front, or back. The zippered sections should be considered the clean area, and the pockets should be considered the working sections.
- Paperwork can carry germs and dust, and should not be carried in the home care bag.
- Nonsterile or exam gloves should be stored in a ziplock or other sealable bag, because loose gloves could tear or become contaminated.
- PPE, which includes isolation gowns, masks, gloves, NIOSH mask, goggles, and disinfectant, should be stored in a large ziplock or other sealable bag inside the zippered (clean) section of the bag.
- Dressings, thermometers, and bandage scissors should be stored inside the zippered (clean) section of the bag.

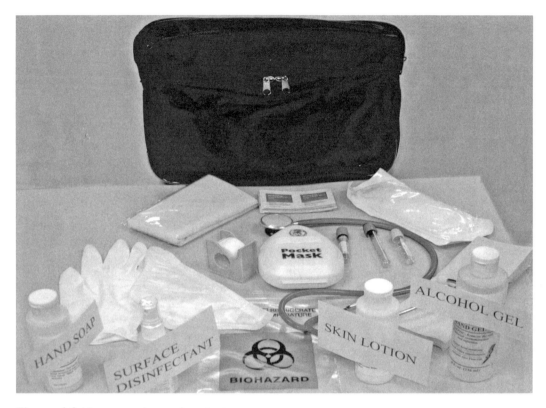

Figure 4-2 Home care bag and contents

- Liquid soap, paper towels, alcohol gel, sphygmomanometer, and other supplies should be kept in the working pockets of the bag for easy access by the home care employee providing client care.

Items restricted from the home care bag/supply box may include:

- Vials of injectables (individual state's departments of pharmacy have guidelines for these vials):
  - Heparin for injection.
  - Saline for injection.
  - Other medications (exception: client labeled/during transport to client's home).
- Expired blood tubes.
- Expired packages of dressings or specialty dressing.
- Saline or other solutions with expired dates.
- Paperwork.
- Torn or damaged packages.
- Nonsafety needles/syringes.
- Contaminated supplies/equipment.
- Mercury thermometers.
- Temperature-sensitive solutions.

Examples of temperature-sensitive solutions are:

- Peroxide (59–86°F).
- Hibiclens (68–77°F).
- Calcium alginate wound products (store in cool, dry area).
- Hand gel (store at room temperature).
- Skin bond (keep away from heat, open flame or sparks).
- Surface disinfectant (store at 50–120°F).

Special handling of these products may be necessary to protect them from temperature extremes. The home care employee should store these products overnight in the home, and during the day should remove the products from direct sunlight. The home care employee designates a clean section of the automobile trunk for client-ready supplies and dressings. A box with a lid is sufficient for this purpose.

Bags of supplies should be closed during storage and transport. Items issued from the home care agency supply room as client ready should be carried into the client's house in an individual clean sturdy bag usually issued by the home care agency. Product expiration dates should be checked often. During transport to the client, these supplies should be stored in the designated clean section of the trunk inside a covered box or closed bag and separated from the dirty section.

Hazardous Waste and Contaminated Items

Lab specimens should be carried in a hard-sided cooler. A small sharps container covered by a ziplock or other sealable plastic bag may fit inside the hard cooler, thus condensing biohazard items into one container for transport. The sealable bag around the sharps container provides added protection from spills.

All hazardous waste generated in the client's home should be disposed of in a safe, efficient manner. All sharps used by agency personnel should be inserted uncapped and intact into a rigid container that is identified with the biomedical hazard sign. Approved sharps containers must be puncture resistant and leakproof on the sides and bottom. The sharps container will be located near the site of the procedure requiring use of sharps. When not prohibited by state law, if left in the client's home, the sharps container will be stored in a safe location appropriate to the home situation. The sharps container should be replaced when two-thirds full.

When the sharps container is removed from the home, the lid should be securely closed. Sharps containers identified with the biomedical hazard logo should not be disposed of in the client's trash. The sharps container should be transported inside an area of the vehicle not occupied by passengers and taken to the collection site at the office.

Thick-walled plastic containers (bleach or detergent bottles), with their lids taped securely in place, may be used to collect client-generated sharps. This type of container may be discarded in the client's trash unless prohibited by local law. In the community where disposal of a client-generated sharps container is prohibited, the local sanitation department should have an alternate disposal procedure, which can be recommended to the client.

Other hazardous materials generated in the home are dressings or materials contaminated with blood/body fluids. Place infected material in the plastic wrapper in which dressings were packaged and place this bag into a plastic bag. Dispose of this bag directly into the waste container outside the client's home and then to the hazardous waste collection site at the agency. Dressings that are dripping blood or other potentially infectious material when squeezed should be placed in a secondary container that is closeable to prevent leakage and labeled or color-coded in red or orange. Red and orange indicate the materials are hazardous wastes. This container is placed in the designated waste-collection site at the agency.

Equipment Cleaning and Biomedical Spills

Contaminated equipment in the home needs to be cleaned to the appropriate level of disinfection. Sterile prepackaged disposable supplies are normally used in home care. Sterile single-use products must not be reused. Products used for cleaning or disinfection of equipment include a bleach solution of one part bleach to nine parts water, 70 percent alcohol, or a commercially prepared surface disinfectant used for hard surface cleaning only. Surface disinfectant is not to be used on porous surfaces, as the solution may be absorbed by porous surfaces and residual disinfectant may cause tissue irritation. Contaminated equipment should be taken to the soiled supply room at the agency as soon as possible after leaving the client's home.

To clean scales used for adult weight, place a disposable plastic barrier bag under the scale prior to placing on the floor. After use, clean with surface disinfectant, and allow the scale to air dry for 10 minutes. To clean a baby scale, place the scale on a table with a safe base and then place a disposable protective cover or pad on the scale. After use, clean with surface disinfectant and allow it to air dry for 10 minutes. Note that *only the baby scales are covered with a protective cover during the weigh process.* Think of the procedure as WEIGH, SPRAY (let dry for 10 minutes) AND STORE! A cleaned scale may be stored in a sturdy plastic bag in the car.

To clean biomedical spills, the home care employee should use PPE as appropriate and the spill kit that is issued by the agency. The cleaning steps are:

- Apply gloves and a gown if needed.
- Use gloved hands and stiff cardboard or the scoop provided in the spill kit to remove broken glass or sharps from the spill area.
- If unable to wash and rinse the area, remove heavy soilage with paper towels.
- Place used paper towels in plastic bag.
- Place sharps/broken glass in sharps container.
- Spray area with hard surface disinfectant. Allow to remain wet for 10 minutes for optimum kill time.
- Wipe area with paper towels, disposing of towels in plastic bag.
- Remove gloves. Dispose of the plastic bag in a trash can and wash your hands.
- For contamination of carpet or fabric, contact agency Infection Control Nurse.

Employee Evaluations

Each employee providing direct client care should receive periodic on-site evaluations in the form of supervisory visits by their clinical supervisor or manager. Specific items related to compliance with infection-control policies will be evaluated. Specific problems should be addressed with the individual employee involved.

The clinical supervisor, manager, or educator may observe the hand hygiene technique of the employee utilizing a luminescent powder or cream and ultraviolet light. This may be done during initial orientation and periodically. This technique provides testing of the effectiveness of the employee's hand hygiene and demonstrates weak areas of hand hygiene.

Client Care Procedures

The home care nurse cares for clients' total needs, which include wound care via dressings; the insertion, care, and irrigation of urinary catheters; administration of intravenous fluids; and enteral feedings. Adherence to the principles of infection control help to prevent wounds, pressure ulcers, irrigation solutions, equipment, and tubes from becoming infected and negatively affecting the client's health.

Wound care in the home can be particularly challenging. Home care nurses provide wound care for surgical wounds, dehisced surgical wounds, decubiti, drains, central lines, and picc lines, and other equipment. Home care nurses should follow the principles of clean or sterile technique as ordered by the physician. Additionally, the use of transmission-based isolation precautions in the presence of multidrug-resistant organisms prevents transmission of these organisms via carriage on the hands or equipment.

The components of clean (medical asepsis) technique include:

- Careful and frequent hand hygiene.
- Wearing sterile gloves to apply sterile dressings.
- Use of unsterile gloves with frequent change of gloves when handling contaminated material (such as soiled dressings).
- Wearing personal protective equipment to avoid direct contact with infectious material.

The components of sterile (surgical asepsis) technique include:

- Washing hands meticulously with antimicrobial soap.
- Using a sterile field.
- Wearing sterile gloves, mask, and gown.

Home care nurses should read the manufacturer's use and storage information prior to utilization of dressing material. For example, packing gauze that is stored dry should never have a solution like normal saline added to the bottle of dry gauze; rather, the packing should be extracted using clean technique and then moistened with the saline.

Prevention of infection in the presence of an indwelling catheter insertion, replacement, and maintenance can be accomplished through:

- The use of a closed system.
- Hand hygiene prior to manipulation of the catheter.
- Maintenance of the catheter below the level of the bladder to prevent reflux.
- Use of sterile technique when changing the catheter.

Long-term self-catheterization clients need to be instructed on procedures to safely clean and reuse their catheters. A procedure for this is included in the client teaching section of this chapter.

Nebulizer tubing and other reusable respiratory equipment are avenues for harboring and transporting infectious organisms, and must be cleaned and disinfected after each use per manufacturer's recommendations.

Infection Reporting

A home care agency's plan and focus for infection surveillance is taught and reviewed with home care employees during their orientation and annually. For consistency, a set of definitions for home care-associated infections should be written for the clinicians to follow when reporting client infections. Definitions combine specific clinical findings with results of laboratory tests to

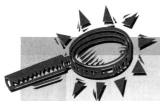

Evidence-Based Practice Box 4-1

"Best-Practice" Approach to Indwelling Urinary Catheters in the Home

A "best-practice" approach has been shown to decrease urinary tract infections (UTIs) in home care clients. Sixteen home care agencies in Arizona participated in a "best-practice" project to monitor and treat urinary tract infections. Participation in the project required developing a standard definition for a UTI, identifying standard indicators for UTIs, developing data collection instruments, establishing guidelines for agency participation, and analyzing data.

Implementation standards for the project were developed by reviewing practice standards and published research articles. Project outcomes were development of a consensus definition of UTI, standard indicators of UTI, and ways to monitor UTIs.

At a large New Jersey agency (services to 10,000 home care clients annually) nurses, as part of a performance improvement review, initiated a catheter management program. The program, which was very similar to the project described above, sought to distinguish through scientific research differences between current practice and "best practice." New standards were developed and initiated that resulted in standardized catheter management, standardized protocol for urine specimen collection, and timely and appropriate urine infection treatment.

(Emr & Ryan, 2004; Long et al., 2002).

form algorithms for determining the presence and classification of infections. A physician's diagnosis of infection is based on direct observations and clinical judgment and is an acceptable criterion for defining an infection when accompanied by an order for antimicrobial therapy.

An infection that is associated with a complication or extension of an infection already present on admission is not considered agency-associated unless a change in pathogen or symptoms indicates a new infection. This information does not alter client treatment, but is necessary for compiling statistical data.

For an infection to be defined as agency-associated there must be no evidence that the infection was present or incubating at the time of admission. Infections that are present or incubating 72 hours or longer where indicated by the specific situation at the time of admission to the agency are non-agency-associated infections.

The home care employee should report infections on an infection-control reporting form, which should contain:

- The client's name.
- Home care start of care date.
- Date of infection.
- Site of infection.

- Organism.
- Antibiotic name, dose, route, frequency, and duration.
- Hospital date, if applicable.
- Symptoms of infection.

The home care employee should also be careful to report to an agency supervisor any employee contagious illness or occupational exposure. Examples of reportable illnesses are conjunctivitis, varicella (chickenpox), varicella zoster (shingles), pertussis, and tuberculosis. The employee health nurse may remove the employee suspected of having a contagious illness from work.

Client Teaching

Clients and their families often misunderstand basic principles of infection control. It is important that the nurse instruct the client and the client's caregiver about infection control. Following verbal instructions, written instructions should be left in the home. Procedures 4-2, 4-3, and 4-4 are sample-teaching sheets of three procedures that are commonly performed by caregivers in the home. The nurse may leave similar instruction sheets in the home for client and/or caregiver review.

Procedure 4-2

Basic Wound Care

Procedure	Rationale
1. Place new dressing packages and gloves and a trash bag near the work area on a clean table.	Close proximity to work area.
2. Wash hands with soap and water for 10 to 20 seconds. Dry well.	Reduces transmission of microorganisms.
3. Open dressing packages, leave dressings sitting in the opened packages.	Sterile dressings remain sterile while in their packages.
4. Put on clean gloves.	Prevents transmission of infectious organisms to hands.
5. Remove soiled dressing followed by used gloves and put them in the trash bag.	Reduces transmission of organisms.

Procedure 4-2 continued

Procedure	Rationale
6. Wash hands and put on clean gloves.	Allows for handling of new dressings.
7. Look at the wound and note redness, odor, and drainage.	Indicates status of wound healing.
8. Clean the wound and put on clean dressings as taught by your home care nurse.	Protects wound.
9. Take off gloves and wash your hands.	Reduces transmission of organisms.
10. Tie the top of the trash bag and place into an outside garbage can.	Reduces transmission of organisms.
11. Record a description of the wound for discussion.	Preserves wound assessment for discussion with home care nurse.

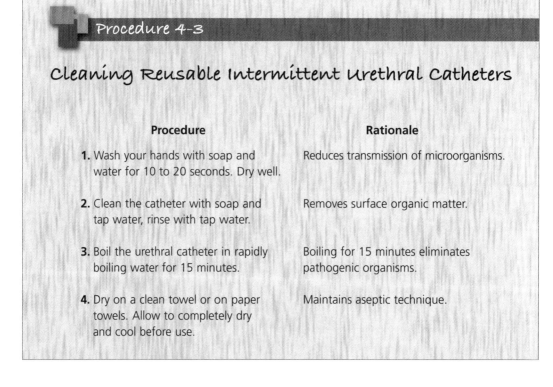

Procedure 4-3

Cleaning Reusable Intermittent Urethral Catheters

Procedure	Rationale
1. Wash your hands with soap and water for 10 to 20 seconds. Dry well.	Reduces transmission of microorganisms.
2. Clean the catheter with soap and tap water, rinse with tap water.	Removes surface organic matter.
3. Boil the urethral catheter in rapidly boiling water for 15 minutes.	Boiling for 15 minutes eliminates pathogenic organisms.
4. Dry on a clean towel or on paper towels. Allow to completely dry and cool before use.	Maintains aseptic technique.

Procedure 4-3 continued

Procedure	Rationale
5. Put cleaned urethral catheters in a new ziplock or similar plastic bag or a clean, closeable container.	Protects catheters from outside environment.
6. Always look at catheters before use. Throw a catheter away that is hard, cracked, or torn.	Assures that defective catheters will not be used.

Procedure 4-4

Standard Infection Control

Procedure	Rationale
1. Wash your hands thoroughly with soap and warm water before and after client care.	Reduces transmission of organisms.
2. Place needles, razors, or other sharp objects used on or by the client in a hard plastic or metal container with a screw on lid. DO NOT USE GLASS. Example: Put the client's insulin needles in an empty liquid laundry detergent bottle.	Prevents sharps from puncturing the sides of the containers and prevents injury. Glass may break.
3. Place used bandages and medical gloves in a tightly closed plastic bag before putting them in the household trash.	Reduces transmission of organisms.
4. Do not place used dressings or dirty linen on countertops or eating surfaces	Used dressings and dirty linen are contaminated.
5. Ask the client with a lung infection or cold to cover his or her mouth and nose when sneezing or coughing.	Reduces transmission of airborne organisms.

Procedure 4-4 continued

Procedure	Rationale
6. Do not share razors, toothbrushes, eating utensils, or drinking glasses with the client.	Reduces transmission of organisms.
7. Wash dishes in hot soapy water and air-dry or use a dishwasher.	Maintains medical asepsis (clean technique).
8. Store dirty linen away from other members of the household. Dirty linen can be washed with regular laundry.	Reduces transmission of organisms.
9. If the client has an infection like MRSA, VRE, or TB ask your doctor or nurse for infection-control advice.	Obtain best possible infection-control advice.

Summary

This chapter discussed infection control in home care with an emphasis on infection-control programs in home care agencies and issues that are of interest to home care employees. The incidence and treatment of selected infectious organisms that home care employees may encounter in the home were identified and discussed. Tools and techniques used for control of infectious organisms in the home, such as personal care equipment and isolation precautions, were described, along with specific procedures aimed at controlling infectious organisms in the home.

The client, home care employee, and home care agency are partners in the goals to prevent the spread of infection and to provide excellent-quality care resulting in positive outcomes. These goals can be accomplished with an understanding of basic infection-control principles and by following the infection-control tools outlined in this chapter.

References

Centers for Disease Control and Prevention (CDC). (2001). *Caring for someone with AIDS at home.* Atlanta: U.S. Department of Health and Human Services:

http://www.cdc.gov/hiv/pubs/BROCHURE/careathome.htm

Centers for Disease Control and Prevention (CDC). (2002a). *Guideline for hand hygiene in health-care settings: Recommendations of the health care infection control practices advisory committee and the HICPAC/SHEA/APIC/IDSA hand hygiene task force. MMWR, 51* (No. RR-16).

Centers for Disease Control and Prevention (CDC). (2002b). *Hand hygiene guidelines fact sheet.* Atlanta: U.S. Department of Health and Human Services:

http://www.cdc.gov/od/oc/media/pressrel/fs021025.htm

Centers for Disease Control and Prevention (CDC). (2003, April 1). *VISA/VRSA–vancomycin-intermediate/resistant Staphylococcus aureus.* Atlanta: U.S. Department of Health and Human Services:

http://www.cdc.gov/ncidod/hip/vanco/VANCO.htm

Centers for Disease Control and Prevention (CDC). (2004a). *Basic information about SARS.* Atlanta: U.S. Department of Health and Human Services:

http://www.cdc.gov/ncidod/sars/factsheet.htm

Centers for Disease Control and Prevention (CDC). (2004b). *Get smart: Know when antibiotics work.* Atlanta: U.S. Department of Health and Human Services:

http://www.cdc.gov/drugresistance/faqs.htm

Centers for Disease Control and Prevention (CDC). (2005a). *Questions and answers about TB.* Atlanta: U.S. Department of Health and Human Services:

http://www.cdc.gov/nchstp/tb/faqs/qa_introduction.htm

Centers for Disease Control and Prevention (CDC). (2005b, March 7). *Pertussis.* Atlanta: U.S. Department of Health and Human Services:

http://www.cdc.gov/ncidod/dbmd/diseaseinfo/pertussis_t.htm

Centers for Disease Control and Prevention (CDC). (2005c, Sept. 28). *Key facts about influenza and the influenza vaccine.* Atlanta: U.S. Department of Health and Human Services: Retrieved October 17, 2005, from

http://www.cdc.gov/flu/keyfacts.htm

Centers for Disease Control and Prevention (CDC): Division of HIV/AIDS Prevention. (2005d). *Basic statistics.* Atlanta: U.S. Department of Health and Human Services:

http://www.cdc.gov/hiv/stats.htm

Centers for Disease Control and Prevention (CDC): National Center for Infectious Diseases. (2005e). *Viral hepatitis B fact sheet.* Atlanta: U.S. Department of Health and Human Services:

http://www.cdc.gov/ncidod/diseases/hepatitis/b/fact.htm

Centers for Disease Control and Prevention (CDC): National Center for Infectious Diseases. (2005f). *Viral hepatitis C.* Atlanta: U.S. Department of Health and Human Services:

http://www.cdc.gov/ncidod/diseases/hepatitis/c/plan/Prev_Control.htm

Centers for Disease Control and Prevention (CDC). (2005g, Sept. 21). *Methicillin-resistant Staphylococcus aureus: information for clinicians.* Atlanta: U.S. Department of Health and Human Services:

http://www.bt.cdc.gov/disasters/hurricanses/katrina/mrsainfoclinicians.asp

Centers for Disease Control and Prevention (CDC). (2005h). *CA-MRSA information for the public.* Atlanta: U.S. Department of Health and Human Services:

http://www.cdc.gov/ncidod/hip/aresist/ca_mrsa_public.htm

Centers for Disease Control and Prevention (CDC). (2005i). *Multidrug-resistant organisms in non-hospital health care settings: Frequently asked questions.* Atlanta: U.S. Department of Health and Humans Services:

http://www.cdc.gov/ncidod/hip/ARESIST/nonhosp.htm

Centers for Disease Control and Prevention (CDC). (2005j). *Treating head lice infestation.* Atlanta: U.S. Department of Health and Human Services:

http://www.cdc.gov/ncidod/dpd/parasites/lice/factsht_head-lice_treating.htm

Centers for Disease Control and Prevention (CDC). (2005k). *Scabies fact sheet.* Atlanta: U.S. Department of Health and Human Services:

http://www.cdc.gov/ncidod/dpd/parasites/scabies/factsht_scabies.htm

DeLaune, S. C., & Ladner, P. K. (2006). *Fundamentals of nursing: Standards and practice* (3rd ed.). Clifton Park, NY: Thomson Delmar Learning.

Emr, K., & Ryan, R. (2004). Best practice for indwelling catheter in the home setting. *Home Healthcare Nurse, 22*(12), 820–830.

Long, C. O., Anderson, C., Greenberg, E. A., & Woomer, N. (2002). Defining and monitoring indwelling catheter-related urinary tract infections. *Home Healthcare Nurse, 20*(4), 255–262.

Maine Department of Human Services, Bureau of Health. (2004). *Pertussis update: Home care of the pertussis patient.*

http://www.maine.gov/dhhs/boh/mip/v-pertussis.html

Rhinehart, E., & McGoldrick, M. M. (2006). *Infection control in home care.* Gaithersburg, MD: Aspen.

World Health Organization. (Jan. 15, 2004). *Avian influenza factsheet.*

http://www.who.int/mediacentre/factsheets/avian_influenza/en/

World Health Organization. (December 9, 2005). *Cumulative number of confirmed human cases of Avian Influenza (H5N1) reported to WHO.*

http://www.who.int/csr/disease/avian_influenza/country/cases_table_/2005_12_09/en/index

Chapter 5

Safety and Environment

Valerie D. George, RN, PhD
Mary Agnes Kendra, RN, PhD, CNS

Key Terms

Antecedent Phase	Geographics	Safety
Environment Props	Recognized Hazards	

Every day, thousands of home care staff, including nurses, home care aides, physical therapists, occupational therapists, social workers, and other providers, make home visits to families who require assistance to manage their health care needs. These providers numbered 748,700 in 2004 (U.S. Department of Labor Bureau of Labor Statistics, 2004). These health care providers come to the specialty with a variety of life experiences, attitudes, beliefs, and values that enable them to function in this dynamic area of practice. However, with the spiralling of violence in society and accompanying violence in the workplace, **safety,** defined as freedom from danger, is a major concern for home care practitioners. This chapter will discuss safety and environment as related to the home care industry. As the demand for home care services increases due to shortened length of stays and an aging population with several chronic diseases, concerns regarding **safety** and freedom from danger become paramount.

Safety in the unstructured environment of home care has been a concern since the inception of this area of specialty practice. Kalish and Kalish (1978) reported that nursing texts as early as the 1890s cautioned public health nurses about how they should dress and their general demeanor to avoid being harassed, being injured, or suffering physical or emotional harm during home visits.

The clinical specialty of home care may be described as involving a high degree of uncertainty and unpredictability (McPhaul & Lipscomb, 2004). Each home visit involves unknown factors, such as the status of the client since the last contact or at the initial contact, the situational context of the home and the community where the client lives, the completeness of the information that has been provided regarding the client's health status and plan of care, and the necessary skills and competencies that will be needed to address the client's needs. Nurses working in this field must understand and appreciate the fact that "minimizing the risk to the worker involves an understanding of the links between the working environment, working practices, and risk" (Patterson, McCornish, & Bradley, 1999, p. 4).

This field is also risky for home care workers because of the many situations encountered in the environment that threaten their personal safety and that of the client and employer (Denton, Zeytinoğhu, & Davies, 2002). Media reports of crime or untoward events in communities, social unrest, and limited experiences working in the home may trigger feelings of apprehension and concern among staff that should be addressed with agency supervisors or administrators. In this chapter we will address factors influencing safety in home care and strategies that the nurse can use to enhance and maintain safety.

Conceptualizing Safety in Home Care

What is safety? Safety can be described as freedom from danger, that is, protection from, or non-exposure to, the risk of injury. It can also be described as trying to minimize harm, injury, or damage. In nursing, the term is generally accepted to mean protecting the client from harm. However, statements from Nursing's Code of Ethics (American Nurses Association, 2001) indicate the all-inclusive nature of the term "safety" for the profession, and clearly indicate the nurse's responsibility for assuring safety not just for the client but also for himself or herself. When caring for clients in home care, a primary objective regarding safety is trying to minimize harm, or injury to self and others. The Code states:

- The nurse promotes, advocates for, and strives to protect the health, safety, and rights of the client.
- **The nurse owes the same duties to self** as to others, including the responsibility to preserve integrity and safety, to maintain competence, and to continue personal and professional growth.

(ANA, 2001.)

The Occupational Safety and Health Act (OSHA) of 1970 states that employers have a duty to provide a work environment for employees that is free from "**recognized hazards** [which are situations that are] likely to cause death or serious physical harm" (OSHA, 2004). Although home care takes place in non-institutionalized settings controlled by clients, employers have an obligation to assure that home visitors are not sent into situations that place them at risk for harm.

Data on workplace violence indicate that health care and social service workers are at great risk for workplace violence. OSHA (2004) identifies several risk factors that threaten workers' safety, two of which are of particular significance for home care: (1) "working alone, often in remote locations, particularly in high-crime settings, with no back-up or means of assistance such as communication devices or alarm systems; and (2) lack of training of staff in recognizing and managing escalating hostile and assaultive behavior" (p. 4). Threats to safety may also result from threatening verbal or nonverbal behavior, sexual harassment, transfer of body fluids or droplets from an infected person, physical exertion that results in straining or injuring the musculoskeletal system, and intimidation or threats with a weapon, object, or dog.

Unlike hospitals, the environment of home care can be characterized as unstructured, fluid, ambiguous, and full of uncertainty. The home care worker often travels to the home alone, and is in a one-to-one relationship with the client and the family. Colleagues are not readily available for discussion of problems that arise or to provide assistance with procedures to be completed. The client and family are the gatekeepers for the home, and nurses must keep in mind that gaining entrance requires negotiation.

Who Makes Home Visits?

Nurses engaged in home care today reflect different levels of education, skills, competencies, experience in the specialty, and work experience. Historically, public health nurses and community health nurses were prepared at the baccalaureate level or had advanced preparation in public health. The curricula of these programs included didactic and clinical experiences that focused on the unique nature of the field, including knowing the community, its structure, key informants, and resources; home visiting; dealing with ambiguity and uncertainty; development of assertiveness and communication skills; ethical and legal components of care; and policies and procedures guiding practice. When those nurses enter the specialty with prior experience in the field, they have less difficulty managing the uncertainty and ambiguity of the practice (Allender & Spradley, 2005). Today, however, many providers have limited preparation in the process of home visiting, and are more focused on the tasks to be performed. Nevertheless, home care workers, regardless of job category, must have a high degree of knowledge, confidence, competence, and skills to provide care skillfully, ethically, and within established guidelines and professional standards. Their knowledge, understanding, and perceptions of the clinical situation influence how they (1) prepare for the visit, (2) safeguard themselves and the client, (3) interpret and implement the client's plan of care, and (4) adhere to agency policies and procedures.

Perception of Safety

Everyone in the course of living experiences threats to safety. When confronted by these situations, the nurse has to recognize the situation as posing a threat, evaluate the type and level of threat, and decide on a course of action to avoid, reduce, or minimize the threat. It must be acknowledged that each nurse's response to threats is individualized and reflects his or her familiarity with risk factors, past experiences dealing with risk factors, propensity toward risk-taking, personal circumstances, time of day, and potential outcome. During this cognitive perceptual process the nurse uses past experiences, available resources, and personal attributes to decide on the course of action (Kendra & George, 2001).

Contributors to Safety

There are four major contributors to safety in home care: the community of the visit, the client, the nurse, and the home care agency. The quality of the relationship among these care components is influenced by personal circumstances of the client and staff member; the client's health status and ability to participate in activities of daily living (ADL) and self-care; staff behavior and attitudes; agency policy and procedures; ethical, legal, and economic issues;

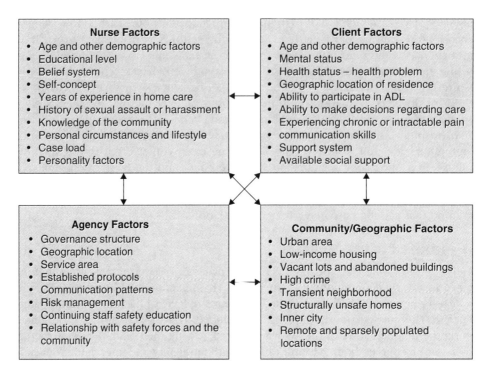

Figure 5-1 Factors influencing perception of and response to threats to safety.

quality of social activities in the community where the client resides and the agency operates; and time of day. Figure 5-1 depicts the interrelationship among these factors.

The personal and situational context of the client influences the client's ability to contribute to safety. The personal and situational context includes attitudes, beliefs, values, attributes, demographics, health status, level of care required, ability to participate in self-care, and availability of a caregiver in the home. Clients who can actively participate in their care, and whose cognitive and psychological status is not diminished, are less likely to experience or participate in behaviors that threaten their safety or that of the nurse. Unfortunately, due to the variety of clients being visited, it is unwise to negate the possibility of any client or family member posing a threat to safety. Nevertheless, to assure a safe environment requires the cooperation and commitment of the client, the nurse, the agency, and involvement of safety forces for law enforcement in the community (Christopher & Beck, 1997; Sylvester & Reisener, 2002).

Home care agencies have established missions, goals, and objectives that provide the framework for how care is provided. The nurse as an agent of the agency (the employer) is expected to fulfill its mission within established parameters and professional judgment. Failure of nurses to practice accordingly exposes both the agency and the nurse to risk (liability). On the other hand, the employer has the responsibility to provide the nurse with the human and material resources necessary to engage in safe practice including personal protection to enhance and promote safety.

If the agency provides service to clients in neighborhoods that have a high crime rate, ethnic unrest, violence, transient tenement houses, and illegal drug use, heightened safety precautions should be implemented to protect workers. Therefore, the agency should give careful consideration to the service areas that it covers to avoid placing staff in danger of harm. Specific policies to promote safety should be developed by agency administrators and staff with input from stake-holders in the community, and reviewed at least annually (Distasio, 2000a).The agency should discuss its safety standards with clients and their families when the contract is initiated.Their understanding and agreement to adhere to them at the outset sets acceptable safety parameters and avoids surprises when problems occur. Clear policies for terminating or refusing to visit a client due to overwhelming risk factors, and use of a buddy system or security escorts in high-risk areas, should be discussed with staff to increase their awareness of these options.

Inherent in OSHA's 2004 guidelines is the employer's responsibility to establish an effective safety promotion program that includes four elements: (1) management commitment and employee involvement, (2) worksite analysis, (3) hazard prevention and control, and (4) safety and health training. Consequently, it is ethically inappropriate to place a worker in a situation with known risk factors without providing sufficient support to protect him or her from harm (Christopher & Beck, 1997; Kendra & George, 2001).

The community where the client resides also plays a significant role in assuring and supporting safety. Communities have resources that promote and provide safety, such as adequate street lighting, buildings in good repair, paved and accessible roads, sidewalks, block watch, visible police presence, housing inspectors, community services such as public transportation, garbage pick-up, snow removal, and animal wardens to control roaming dogs. Risk factors can also be objectively assessed by accessing data from the 2000 U.S. Census for the particular community. This data includes information related to population, demographics, income level, educational level, and type of industry for each community.

A community assessment, done by the agency, provides the agency's workforce with information related to safety forces, rate of violent crimes, and frequency of fires. Additional information about the community can be obtained from the Centers for Disease Control and Prevention's (CDC) website at http://www.cdc.gov, and the local chamber of commerce. These resources enable the nurse to develop a comprehensive picture of the community and its assets and hazards that threaten safety from an environmental, physical, bacteriological, and mechanical perspective.

Phases of the Home Visit

Making a home visit involves four distinct phases: (1) the **antecedent phase,** which involves preparing for the visit (Byrd, 1995); (2) getting to the home from the agency; (3) being in the home; and (4) leaving the home and returning to the agency. Attention to the dynamics of these phases enables the nurse to gain an appreciation of the client situation and develop deliberative responses to achieve established goals and objectives. Each phase of the home visit is discussed below.

Phase 1: Antecedent Phase

The antecedent phase of the home visit involves the nurse in the process of preplanning, wherein he or she considers the environmental context; the client; personal knowledge, skills, and competencies; and agency factors; and asks questions to assure safety during each of these phases. Thus, prior to visiting a client, it is in the nurse's best interest to have as much information as possible about the geography of where the client lives, the diagnosis(es), family composition, physicians' names and phone numbers, and the name of the caregiver. These pieces of information are vital for framing responses to situations encountered during the process of home visiting to assure that responses and decisions reflect the best interest of the client, and perhaps more importantly, minimize risk to the nurse. The goal of this phase is to develop awareness of the client being visited, the specific health concern, the available and necessary resources for care, and the situational context of the visit. Box 5-1 identifies some of the specific areas that the nurse should consider as the home visit is being planned, and presents important questions that the nurse should consider during the planning process.

BOX 5-1 ANTECEDENT PHASE: PREPLANNING SAFETY ASSESSMENT FOR HOME VISITS

Environmental Assessment
- Where is the client's home located?
- How many miles from the agency?
- What do you know about that community or neighborhood?
- What method of transportation will you use to travel to the client's home?
- What is the weather report for today?
- Are there any media reports of activities in the client's community or along the route that pose a possible threat to safety?
- Are safety forces readily available?

Client Assessment
- Who is the client?
- What is her or her medical diagnosis?
- What is his or her nursing diagnosis?
- What level or type of care is required?
- How long has the client had this health problem?
- What type of nursing care is required?
- Does the client have the necessary information, supplies, and equipment for the care required?
- Can the client assist with activities of daily living?
- Are there other family members in the home or readily accessible to assist with client care?

Nurse's Self-Assessment
- Do I have the requisite knowledge, skills, and competencies to care for this client?
- What additional information do I need to care for this client?
- What type of equipment is in the home or will be needed to provide care?
- What agency policies and procedures will I enact during this visit?
- Who can I call on for assistance in case of an emergency?
- Do I have any personal concerns that may prevent me from carrying out the client's plan of care?

Box 5-1 continued

Agency Assessment

- Are nurses' concerns about situations that pose risk acknowledged by the agency?
- What is the agency policy regarding "buddy systems" or police escorts? Are they provided when requested or based on the risk factors in communities visited?
- What is the process of reporting situations or incidents that threaten safety? Is there an incident report form? Where is it kept? How often is it used?
- What are the policies and procedures for dealing with violence and other threats to safety when they occur?
- What kind of support does the agency provide if the nurse experiences a threatening incident?
- Does the agency have a working relationship with safety forces for law enforcement in the community being visited, so that staff in the field can call on them as required?
- What is the process for reporting adverse clinical situations of the client to the primary care provider?
- What is the policy regarding the nurses' ability to refuse visits?
- Does the agency provide and pay for cell phones or pagers?
- Is there a safety committee?
- What information is available regarding threats to safety experienced by members of the staff visiting in client neighborhoods?
- What type of safety information is provided about various neighborhoods that nurses visit?

Phase 2: Getting to the Client's Home

Getting to the home from the home care agency requires assessment of the environment, client, nurses and agency.

Environmental Assessment   The environment of the home visit includes factors external to and within the home. **Geographics** refer to the environmental context of the location in which the visit occurs. How home visitors perceive the geographics of the visit is influenced by their knowledge and familiarity with the area, their orientation to the various communities, the visibility of police, media reports of incidents of safety hazards, their perception of the situational context of the visit, and the availability of **environmental props.** Environmental props refer to factors in the environment that can be used to protect home care workers from harm. In large and small cities the worker has to be aware of threats to personal safety posed by inadequately maintained buildings, abandoned houses, vacant lots strewn with trash, and people hanging out in doorways, on the streets, and in hallways. These factors must be viewed from the perspective of the home visitor and the geographical areas that must be traversed to travel from the agency (Fazzone et al., 2000). For example, workers

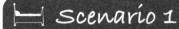

Scenario 1

Inclement Weather Conditions

When you leave the client's home, you notice that snow is falling heavily, and as you get about a mile away, you see that the road is becoming impassable. You remember that the tires on your car are worn. In addition, you do not have access to your cell phone, as it died earlier in the day. What would you do?

Stay in your car as the road seems impassable.
Go back to the client's home.
Continue on your trip back to the agency.

What type(s) of risk(s) are you dealing with in the above options?

may travel to residences within the city limits, or between the city and the suburbs or to rural areas. Some workers may travel in rural areas where there are long distances between homes, while others may travel to remote locations over hazardous terrains. These situations pose a threat to safety because the nurse may have difficulty alerting neighbors that he or she is in danger and needs assistance. Thus, having a working cell phone or a communication device is an important safety measure—your "life-line."

Seasonal variations also create threats to the workers' safety—winter weather with ice, sleet, snow, and snowdrifts predisposes to automobile accidents, getting stuck in a snowbank, or skidding. Spring brings flooding, which may make roads impassable. Driving in underpopulated areas for long distances predisposes to fatigue, which lowers response time to hazards encountered while driving (Fazzone et al., 2000; Gellner et al., 1994).

Although it may be difficult to identify which phase is the most important, thinking about getting to the home, for some, may be the most influential factor that determines the ease with which the home visit is conducted. Knowledge of the area, whether based on personal experience or media reports, often conjures up in one's mind that "I am going to a really unsafe area"—even before getting into the car.

More than likely, the nurse will minimize conversation, hoping to get in and out of the home as fast as possible (Kendra et al., 1996). Under these circumstances, if the nurse feels unsafe, it will be difficult to provide good nursing care. Such feelings should be discussed with nursing management.

While traveling, home care workers should look for environmental props. Props may be the police, religious leaders, groups or organizations of people (such as Neighborhood Watch), structures (houses, hospitals, churches, schools, highway guardrails, highway exits), inanimate objects (the car, car horn, whistle, bell, trees and shrubs, streetlights), and postal workers. These props provide shelter, a place to hide, increase visibility, or sound an alarm to alert others that you are in danger.

Home care workers should possess a map of the city in which they work, either purchased or downloaded from the Internet, that charts the directions from the agency to the home of each client to be visited and to those clients in between. Workers who use their vehicles should be sure their cars are in good repair, begin each day with a full tank of gas, and periodically check the gas gauge. When using public transportation, it is wise to have the exact change or

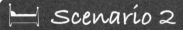

Scenario 2

Geographics Related to Drug Area

You have been asked to visit a client in an area of town that you know has a reputation for having many drug sales on various street corners. When looking at the address, you realize that the client you are supposed to visit is located near one of these corners. As you approach the area in your car, you notice two groups of men standing around telephone booths located on the corners of the intersection where your client's apartment building is located. A couple members of each group seem to be "look-out" persons.

What would you do?
What type(s) of risk(s) are you dealing with here?

a bus or train pass. If possible, the times for client visits should be coordinated with current bus or train schedules to avoid waiting a long time alone at an isolated bus stop or train station. Avoid walking long distances from the bus stop to the client's home; and when walking, walk briskly and purposefully. Directions, when needed, should be sought from a uniformed police officer or firefighter; at a police, fire, or gas station, a supermarket, or a barbershop.

The media provide a valuable service by bringing news of neighborhood events to the public's attention. Home care workers can keep informed about the happenings in the neighborhoods that they visit through radio, television, and newspapers. Other nurses also have information regarding events in the agency's service area. Agencies may post community risk factors on bulletin boards. Rumor verification is necessary, as some people exaggerate negative events while others minimize them. Knowledge of facts from a reliable source avoids undue concern about rumors.

If a client lives in a high-crime area or a "bad neighborhood," it is best to schedule visits in the morning to minimize the risk of contact with gang members, drug traffickers, or people just "hanging out." Nursing management may assist in developing a buddy system or in assigning a security escort for visiting in these areas. Many agencies have arrangements with police departments to provide security for staff and to provide safety information on a regular basis regarding the community. Preplanning is an important component of preparedness, but the planning is only as good as the information that is available (Denton et al., 2002; Morris, Krueger, & Yaross, 2004; Paterson et al., 1999; Sylvester & Reisener, 2002). Nurses still have the obligation to be aware of the risks and exercise caution and good judgment as they navigate the different environments where clients reside.

Client Assessment   The practice of home care focuses on providing safe care to clients regardless of age, gender, ethnicity, belief system, health status or socioeconomic status. Planning to promote safety requires the same care whether the nurse is planning an initial or follow-up visit, or when the nurse makes his or her first home visit. The basic client assessment identified in Box 5-1 provides a holistic framework that contributes to safety. The answers to the open-ended question "Who is the client?" provide information regarding demographics, health problems, level and type of care required, the client's ability to participate in self-care, and the availability of family caregivers. The assessment also highlights potential threats to safety.

Client data may reveal potential threats related to the following factors. An example of each is given.

1. Physical-biochemical—nurse exposure to body fluids from wounds in different stages of healing.

2. Mechanical—client is bedridden and weighs 279 pounds.

3. Cognitive-emotional—client has frequent mood swings and periods of combativeness.

4. Interpersonal-relational—client's primary caretaker, a daughter, was arrested at the home two nights ago on a charge of domestic violence and elder abuse.

5. Valuative-attitudinal—client is a primipara, two days postpartum, who is having difficulty with breast-feeding.

6. Financial—client has three children under the age of four years whose height and weight are below the mean for their age; the children are also anemic.

7. Sociocultural—client reports that he is "a prisoner" in his home due to poor vision because of his inability to drive to the local senior center. (Antonovsky, 1979, 1984.)

Risky Diagnoses   There are certain diseases that pose risks to the nurse providing health care. These diseases, which are of a physical-biochemical nature, communicable or infectious, include tuberculosis, hepatitis B, and HIV/AIDS. Preplanning to assure strict adherence to standard precautions in all aspects of the care process protects the client, nurse, members of the household, and community from infection. The client and family members must be taught about body fluid precautions to reduce the possibility of transfer of infection. For example, the client diagnosed with tuberculosis who has positive sputum must be taught about the spread of the disease and how to follow certain procedures such as coughing and sneezing into tissues and the importance of frequent hand-washing.

When visiting a client with a communicable or infectious condition, or a possibility of such, the nurse should always use personal protective equipment (mask, gown, and gloves) to prevent disease transmission, and should also review standard precautions with the client and family members. The home environment should be observed for signs of compliance. The importance of having and using personal protective equipment is imperative. If in doubt, use the equipment. Refer to Chapter 4 for information on communicable diseases and personal protective equipment.

Supplies and Equipment   Are needed supplies and equipment available in the home? In hospital settings, supplies and equipment are readily available to provide care. If the nurse needs assistance from staff to care for a client, colleagues are readily available to assist. In the home setting, staff is not available to assist unless the home care agency uses the buddy system; in addition, supplies and equipment may not be immediately available. Furthermore, supplies and equipment may be plentiful; however, staff may not be available due to the nature of the visit. In addition, the client may live alone, or the family caregivers may not want to or may be unable to assist with ambulation, dressing changes, or monitoring body processes (such as intake, output, and frequency of bowel elimination). These limitations have potential for complicating the client's plan of care and threatening safety unless the nurse anticipates and plans for them in advance.

Ergonomics   A client's inability to move or transfer without assistance demands that the nurse use good body mechanics and assistive devices appropriately to prevent the client from falling and to avoid ergonomic insults that cause back or shoulder injuries to the nurse. Nurses are

Scenario 3

No Supplies for Dressing Change

You arrive at a home, enter the house, and after assessing the client situation begin to prepare for providing nursing care. Today, your nursing intervention involves changing a dressing to a leg ulcer. You set up for the dressing change and ask the client/caregiver for the additional supplies. You are told that they used the last ones yesterday and the new shipment has not arrived yet. How would you handle this situation?

What would you say to the client?
What would you say to the caregiver?
What would you tell your supervisor?
What type(s) of risk(s) are you dealing with here?

prone to trip due to uneven flooring, scatter rugs, and slippery flooring. These incidents may result in strains, sprains, bruises, and pain in the shoulders, neck, and lower back. In health care workers, back injuries, frequently caused by overexertion, occur 4.5 times more often than in any other type of worker (U.S. Department of Labor, Bureau of Labor Statistics, 2001).

Medications   Cognitively impaired, emotionally distressed, and older adults are prone to medication errors arising from taking prescriptions from multiple providers, taking more than four medications every day, difficulty following complex regimens for a prescription, forgetting to take the medications, not taking medications as ordered, and taking the wrong medication. Medication errors are prone to occur when clients, especially the elderly, take several medications during the day. Numerous prescribed medications increase the risk of drug interactions among elders, many of whom have two or more chronic diseases that require taking very powerful combinations of drugs. Review of the client's record includes an assessment of the number of medications being taken, the schedule for each, how long they have been prescribed, and their intended therapeutic effectiveness (Ellenbecker, Frazier, & Verney, 2004; Miller, 2004).

Scenario 4

Overweight Client

A remarkably overweight client (weighing 350 pounds [DG1]) requests that you transfer him to his wheelchair. The caregiver who is usually present in the home to help you with this transfer has just left to go to the grocery store.

What would you do first?
Then what would you do?
What would to say to the client?
What type(s) of risk(s) are you dealing with?

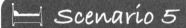

Scenario 5

Teaching the Caregiver

You visit a client who recently was discharged with multiple new medications in addition to the ones she was taking prior to hospitalization. The caregiver (her husband) tells you the medication schedule that he was taught in the hospital. When you make a couple of suggestions that you believe would be helpful, he responds by saying "that's the way they taught me. Why would I want to do anything that would harm my wife? You are only a student—what do you know?"

What would be your first response?
Then what would you do?
What type(s) of risk(s) are you dealing with here?

The nurse should also review and plan to evaluate the medication regimen with the client and family to promote safety. To avoid error, the nurse needs to work with family caregivers to develop a system to minimize possible interactions. When a client complains of tiredness, tachycardia, dyspepsia, headache, thirst, dry skin, constipation, urticaria, frequent urination and/or bowel elimination, one might suspect that untoward interactions of medications are already being manifested. Teaching a client and caregiver about medications and adverse reactions is one of the most important roles of the nurse in making home visits.

In the home setting, the time for the visit must be negotiated or access may be denied. Clients have particular routines that they use to support their life-style. The client may want to watch television, talk on the phone, or listen to music. Caregivers may be too involved, or not involved enough, in what you are trying to do for the client. Visitors may come and leave while you are in the home, disrupting your ability to effectively carry out the client's plan of care.

Scenario 6

Coping with a New Diagnosis

The first visit you have to make is to a 56-year-old client who is newly diagnosed with diabetes (IDDM). She reports that her 7 A.M. glucose reading was 200 (prior to eating breakfast). She is very pleased with this result. You also remember reading that the referral stated that she was a known IV drug user and was finding it very difficult to accept the fact that she has diabetes.

How would you handle this situation to avoid overt (or covert) confrontation?
What are some possible approaches that you can use to reframe her reality about the blood glucose reading?
What type(s) of risk(s) are you dealing with here?

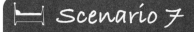

Scenario 7

Inebriated Caregiver

You are assigned to make a visit to a remote area of the county. You forgot your cell phone charger and your cell phone died. The husband comes to the door and has a smell of alcohol on his breath, speaks in slurred voice, and is unsteady in gait. You are to care for his wife, who was discharged four days ago following a right mastectomy.

What would you do first? Why?
What type(s) of risk(s) are you dealing with here?

Pets   Research suggests that pets provide comfort and security to clients (Castelli, Hart, & Zasloff, 2001; Jennings, 1997; Sable, 1995). Although this association is thought to be good for clients, an unruly pet may pose danger to the nurse coming into the home, especially if the client is unable to manage the pet. Additionally, the pet may not be friendly or may cause an allergic reaction. Again, this safety issue is one that needs to be addressed with the client. Often the pet can be placed in another room while care is being provided. If no resolution is achieved to the nurse's satisfaction, then the nursing supervisor needs to be informed and a solution sought within the family context.

Nurse Self-Assessment   The nurse comes to home care with a multitude of life experiences that influence perceptions of the client and the clinical situation. Each nurse has beliefs, values, and attitudes that are different based on culture, ethnicity, age, socioeconomic status, educational level, and personal circumstances. Figure 5-1 identifies some of the factors that influence how nurses view and respond to issues in the clinical situation. These factors contribute to the nurse's overall perception of the frequency with which they experience threats to safety, the degree or level of threat experienced, and their response to threats. A central component of perception is uncertainty regarding a situation or event (Rowe, 1977). Several authors contend that perception and cognition of threats to safety result from how people view the world and their place in it (Antonovsky, 1979, 1984; Kendra & George, 2001; Lazarus, 1966, 1991; Lazarus & Folkman, 1984).

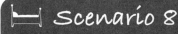

Scenario 8

Dealing with Pets

Upon reviewing the chart, you note that there are two cats and one dog, a collie named Princess, in the home. There is no mention of the behavior of these pets with strangers. You have an allergy to cats.

What would you do first? Why?
What type(s) of risk(s) are you dealing with here?

As the nurse prepares for the visit ("going to see the client"), he or she may have personal concerns regarding the location of the visit, the type and level of care required, the number of visits to be made, and the timeframe for completing the assigned cases (Byrd, 1995). These factors may engender feelings of anxiety, causing the nurse to feel overwhelmed by the enormity of the demands that day. Fazzone and associates (2000) report that organizational and administrative issues, as well as mergers and acquisitions, increased the amount of pressure placed on staff to be more cost-effective and competitive, resulting in higher caseloads and less regard for personal safety. These authors identified the following seven major factors influencing safety of home care staff: (1) unsafe conditions that direct care staff must face; (2) organizational and administrative issues that impede or promote the personal safety of staff; (3) ethical issues staff face daily; (4) protective factors associated with maintaining safety; (5) issues of gender, race, age, and experience; (6) education and training; (7) the potential impact that staff's fear of interpersonal and community violence can have on client care and client outcomes. These pieces of information are vital to facilitate collaboration, coordination, and continuity of care, and to assure that responses and decisions reflect the best interest of clients, and perhaps more importantly, minimize risk to home care staff.

In reviewing the client's record, the types and level of nursing interventions required by the plan of care, and the requisite competencies are reviewed. Box 5-1 poses sample questions that may be considered in a "nurse self-assessment." Nurses may cull appropriate answers from their previous nursing experiences. Additional information is available from colleagues and from resources such as textbooks, research articles, agency policy and procedure manuals, the Internet, and the primary care provider. New or unfamiliar procedures should be reviewed prior to the client visit. In addition, consider taking written instructions and supplementary teaching material for the client.

If prior experiences with the client or family members cause the nurse to feel uncomfortable or uncertain regarding what will transpire at the upcoming visit, these concerns should be explored with the appropriate supervisor. In these discussions, it is prudent to be specific regarding what transpired between the home care worker and the client or family member. Topics for discussion should include the nature of the conflict or situation, the resolution effectiveness of the situation, and remaining or outstanding issues to be resolved. When staff feel threatened by experiences in the home, they will shorten the visit to avoid the possibility of additional harm to themselves (Fazzone et al., 2000; Feldman, Sapienza, & Kane, 1990; Kendra, 1996). When a home care worker is confronted with an uncomfortable situation, it is always appropriate to explore the possibility of providing an escort or a second staff member to accompany the primary worker.

Several studies have explored nurses' perceptions and experiences with risky situations in home care and contend that a variety of factors intersect to increase the possibility of threats to safety (Fazzone et al., 2000; Kendra, 1996). Steinberg (1994) suggests that nurses working in suburban areas in Canada reported fewer incidents of threats than those in urban settings. In addition, clear agency policies, realistic expectations placed on the nurse, a "call-in" system, and the amount of information provided on each client greatly reduced the nurse's perception of being at risk.

Beech (2001) reports that student nurses are at greatest risk of being victims of aggression and violence due to lack of experience in the field and failure of educational programs to provide training on self-defense and management of aggression and violent behavior. Thus, it is important for all home care workers, including students, to keep the aforementioned suggestions uppermost in their thoughts while making home visits, thereby minimizing risk to self, client, and agency.

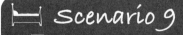

Scenario 9

Sexual Harassment

You are assigned to visit a client to assess her cardiac status. During the visit, her daughter makes inappropriate comments about how nice you look and that she really would like to have a date with you. She asks for your phone number so that she can contact you later that evening. You tell her that it is inappropriate to give home phone numbers to families. When you complete your visits for the day, the daughter is in the school parking lot and approaches you about going out to a local bar. You tell her that you have a girlfriend and refuse her invitation. Two days later, there is a knock at your door, and upon looking through the peep-hole, you see this same person outside your door.

How would you handle this situation?
What type(s) of risk(s) are you dealing with here?

Agency Assessment   The fourth contributor to safety in home care is the agency or organization that provides services to clients in their homes. Regardless of its governance structure, mission, philosophy, and goals, the agency has a dual obligation to provide safe care to clients and to protect the health and safety of its workers. In preparing to visit a client, the nurse should know the policies and procedures that enhance and maintain safety for the client and the nurse as well as guidelines for responding to threats to safety. Box 5-1 identifies important questions related to agency responsibilities that should be considered when planning a home visit.

Although the workplace in home care is the client's home, employers have the obligation to protect their employees from hazards. The General Duty Clause (29USC 1900 5 [a] [1])

Scenario 10

Agency Policies—School and Agency

A group of nursing students who are in the home health nursing course are talking among themselves about going out in twos, which is school policy, versus going out individually. They feel that they are adults, and based upon their academic status in the program, that they can handle "anything" by themselves, and therefore they see no need for the twos rule.

How may they be compromising the agency, the school, and themselves?
What are some of the consequences of following through with their plan?
What type(s) of risk(s) are you dealing with here?

issued by OSHA (1998) states that employers have a "general duty to provide their employees with a workplace free from recognized hazards likely to cause death or serious harm." What are recognized hazards? Any act, incident, or situation that poses a threat to people physically, emotionally, socially, economically, or spiritually. Examples include aggressive verbal or physical behavior from clients or co-workers; pushing, slapping, and scratching; threatening animals; gangs; illegal drug activity in public view; unsafe structures; visiting at night in transient or "bad" neighborhoods without an escort; sexual, ethnic, or religious remarks to intimidate or demean someone; random acts of violence, drive-by shooting, car-jacking, stabbing, and robbery; and sexual harassment by physical contact or verbal expression and rape (Christopher & Beck, 1997; Sylvester & Reisener, 2002).

The agency cannot protect the nurse from every possible threat; however, it can develop and implement specific strategies such as (1) an initial orientation program that addresses various aspects of personal safety; (2) a safety program that involves all levels of staff at the agency and police and fire departments from the community to establish open lines of communication; (3) use of personal protective devices for nurses to limit risk factors; (4) defined services that are periodically evaluated for risk factors; (5) enabling nurses to use their professional judgment to refuse visiting a client if he or she feels that the situation is unsafe; and (6) an ongoing continuing education program that addresses personal safety and provides opportunities for staff to relate their experiences (Christopher & Beck, 1997; Morris et al., 2004; OSHA, 1970; Sylvester & Reisener, 2002).

Nurses should be coached to sharpen their observational and perceptual skills to recognize potential risk factors. Role playing and vignettes are excellent teaching strategies to enhance this process. A survey while driving through a neighborhood or community is a fundamental strategy for identifying potential hazards. Oftentimes, threats occur during one-to-one interactions with clients; thus home care agencies often offer classes and exercises that teach home care personnel how to use nonviolent responses and conflict resolution techniques to prevent a situation from becoming violent (Sitzman, 2001; USDHHS, 1996). The use, care, and maintenance of personal protective equipment and adherence to universal precautions, and adherence to agency policy and procedures, are essential components of safety preparedness.

Home care agencies are providing care to a diverse group of clients requiring primary, secondary, and tertiary care. Nurses are expected to be competent in using multiple and often high-tech procedures to provide care. As a result of the increased emphasis on assuring that the skill mix is appropriate to deliver the required care, more time is spent in competency skills testing of health care workers. Although this aspect is deemed necessary for maintaining agency standards to receive third-party reimbursement, the amount of time devoted toward helping workers deal with situations that pose interpersonal safety risks becomes compromised.

The previous phases presented scenarios that posed problems that might be considered easy to resolve. Unfortunately, there are other areas such as verbal assault, obvious signs of drug use/misuse, unsafe housing, weapons in sight, clients demanding services that are not in their plan of care, or caregiver abuse that will test the nurse's ability to manage the situation. There may be policies and procedures in place by the agency to help nurses define their responsibility in these situations; but again, it is up to the nurse to carefully assess each situation. Open discussion with management is imperative to explore possible options.

Phase 3: Making the Home Visit

In the previous section, assessments that the nurse performs to anticipate and plan for responding to threats to safety during home visits were discussed. However, it is not until the nurse visits the client's home and performs the initial assessment that he or she is able

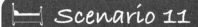

Scenario 11

Weapons—Guns

You enter the home and are escorted to the client's bedroom. Mr. T. has a history of **TIAs**, and most recently has suffered a significant **CVA** with left-sided paralysis. The client's first response is "boy, if I had a gun I'd shoot myself." You look around the room and notice that the top drawer of his bedside stand is partially open, revealing what appears to be a small, loaded revolver.

How would you handle this situation?
What type(s) of risk(s) are you dealing with here?

to ascertain and validate the client's health status and if the desired outcomes are to be achieved. Upon arriving at the client's home, the nurse should feel confident that he or she is prepared to respond to threats encountered during the visit, and that resources are available from the agency or the community to assist if necessary. The nurse also determines what the client and the caregiver know about the health problem, the performance of interventions, and the desired outcomes.

Consider the client situation: What does the nurse know about the client? Reflect on the items in Box 5-1. Are there potential safety threats to the nurse, client, and family members or the agency? At this time, the environment of the home is evaluated for potential threats to the client's safety. Areas of potential danger include stairs and scatter rugs; non-working phones, refrigerators, and stoves; and, at times, family caregivers. Who is in the home and what is their role? If there is an emergency, how and where will you exit the home?

Activities of Daily Living   Many home care clients have difficulty performing activities of daily living, such as bathing, transferring, walking, and moving up or down in bed as would be the case with a client who is comatose. Most nurses have been taught body mechanics in structured settings, unlike home settings, that included beds (or other adjustable apparatus)

Scenario 12

Pets/Dogs

You approach a home, knock on the door, and hear the **LOUD** barking of at least one dog. You remember being bitten by a dog earlier in your life, and it was quite physically and emotionally painful. The husband comes to the door and invites you to come in.

What would be your first response?
Then what would you do?
What types(s) of risk(s) are you dealing with here?

that could be raised or lowered to facilitate ease in providing care. There may have been other items for ambulating clients that will not be available in the home setting, such as a waist belt, lifts, or siderails. The nurse must avoid back injuries when there is not another person in the home to assist with ambulating or transferring clients from bed to a chair. Nurses must remember that protecting the back is of utmost importance in present situations, but more importantly in the future. Back injuries are not easily corrected, and if they are, the chance of reinjuring the area is high based upon the nature of nursing practice. Many back injuries result from overexertion while lifting, pushing, and pulling. These injuries, along with accidental slips, trips, and falls, can result in sprains, strains, hernias, and lower back pain (OSHA, 2004).

Home Conditions   The amount of light in the home may hinder the nurse's ability to assess the client's health status, such as the stage of wound healing and skin color. As a result, the responsibility for controlling the environment to provide safe nursing care has the potential to influence the way in which work will begin. Creation of a clean environment to provide wound care may become a challenge. Other concerns may surface as the home visit continues.

Another home concern is "creepy crawlies"—cockroaches, ants, and other insects that may be visible. Although these insects may be common in the client's house, the nurse may be concerned that they might become members of his or her own home. More often than not, clients are not happy about these insects either, but generally, infestations are due to circumstances beyond their control because they may live in an apartment where the landlord does not provide extermination services. Or, if the client owns the home, financial resources may be insufficient to hire an exterminator. Under such circumstances, it is wise to avoid sitting on upholstered chairs or sofas; it is better to sit on a wooden or metal kitchen chair or just stand and conduct the visit. If neither is available, the client may ask the nurse to sit on an upholstered chair or couch. Responses of refusal should be framed in a way that avoids making clients uncomfortable about their living situation.

There may be situations where the insects or rodents pose a danger to the client's health, such as dressing supplies being "invaded," making sterile dressings impossible to maintain. It is important to discuss concerns with the appropriate supervisor, as the local health department's division of housing may need to be contacted.

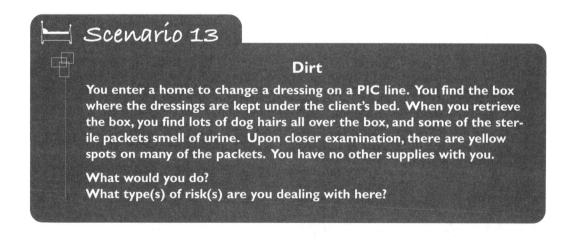

⊨ Scenario 13

Dirt

You enter a home to change a dressing on a **PIC** line. You find the box where the dressings are kept under the client's bed. When you retrieve the box, you find lots of dog hairs all over the box, and some of the sterile packets smell of urine. Upon closer examination, there are yellow spots on many of the packets. You have no other supplies with you.

What would you do?
What type(s) of risk(s) are you dealing with here?

There are home environments that, regardless of the geographical area (urban, suburban, or rural), may appear to be safe from the outside in terms of driving to the home. However, once inside, another picture emerges. Cleanliness, or more accurately, the lack of cleanliness may become a huge concern. Clutter, dirt, and grime on the furniture, and obvious dust or dirt on the floor, tables, windows, and walls may be of concern. Food particles, food containers with spoiled food, and fecal material from numerous pets (or even just one pet), heighten concern that the condition of the home environment compromises the client's health status. The client's bedding may be soiled, and a foul odor may come from the only available bathroom in the home. This situation requires immediate attention. Nurses must consider their role in addressing this situation.

Discussion of these conditions with the client and caregiver is necessary to determine how they plan on cleaning the home. Depending on the resources at their disposal, referral to community agencies may be an option if the client meets eligibility requirements.

At the conclusion of the visit, the nurse should reflect on any potential threats to safety observed and whether they were brought to the attention of the client or caregiver. Were they corrected, or did the client discuss plans for correcting them? What was the response? Was the situation such that a referral to a community agency is needed? Discussions on situations such as these often provide an excellent opportunity for teaching and for reinforcing prior teaching.

Phase 4: Leaving the Home and Returning to the Agency

The primary safety concerns after visiting the client's home relate to documentation of threats to safety of the client and the nurse. Documentation of adverse events that happened between the nurse and the client or members of the client's household should be reported and recorded following agency policy and procedures. The details of the event should be written in the client's medical record and the referring physician or agency notified. Failure to report a threat to safety is a breech of professional ethics and exposes the client, family members, other nurses, and the agency to risk.

The client's need for additional resources to live safely in the home is often a concern for nurses. For example, the nurse observes a change in the client's personal appearance, the kitchen sink and table are stacked with dirty dishes, and the bedroom linen is soiled with body secretions. The client mentions that the caregiver had a death in the family and will be away for two more weeks and that she is barely managing. There is need for intervention.

After the visit may be the time for the nurse to reflect on how the visit was managed; possible threats to safety; the success or lack of success with the interaction; the nurse's feelings of apprehension;, observations related to hearing, smelling, and feeling; and an examination of interactive techniques such as the use of eye contact and voice control.

The nurse may need to review whether the necessary resources to provide care were available, whether the previsit information about the client was accurate, and how perceptions of the client changed over the course of the visit. A last reflection would be: were new insights gained regarding safety?

The Threat of Violence

Distasio (2000a) maintains that violence is a process that spans a continuum with three stages: the baseline stage (during which the person is calm), the pre-assaultive stage (during which the person displays behaviors indicative of altered physical or emotional distress), and the assaultive stage (during which the person exhibits acute excitement, or acts out).

During the pre-assaultive stage, the client displays five behavioral changes: (1) a change in affect evidenced by pressured speech pattern (loud, cursing, shouting, argumentative, threatening); (2) motor agitation evidenced by restlessness, pacing, obstinance; (3) sudden changes in level of consciousness; (4) increased confusion or disorientation; and (5) generalized symptoms such as rapid respiration, enraged facial expression, flaring of the nostrils, clenched fists, reddened face, dilated pupils, and gritting of the teeth indicative of poor tolerance to stress. If any of these behaviors are exhibited by clients during a home visit, the nurse should leave the home immediately.

In today's home care environment, the caseload of many agencies includes clients with behavioral health problems who need counseling and medication management. The following scenario illustrates a home visit by a nurse where violence is suspected.

One of the clients that the nurse is visiting today was discharged from the hospital two weeks ago with the discharge diagnosis of bipolar disorder. The nurse arrives at the home and greets the client and his wife. Nursing intervention for this visit involves monitoring the client's behavior and assessing compliance with his medication regimen. The client directs the nurse to a seat in the living room. His wife sits at the kitchen table with her hands covering her face and appears to be crying. The client frequently looks at her, hits his right thigh with his fist, and sighs loudly. Ten minutes into the visit the client stands up suddenly, and walks toward the kitchen. His wife gets up from the chair immediately, walks toward the nurse and hands him a crumpled piece of paper with the words "HELP ME" scribbled on it. She returns to the kitchen without saying anything to the nurse. The nurse notes that her face appears "puffy" and that there are bruises on her left cheek and scratch marks on her arms. Soon the client returns to the room with his meds and explains how he takes each of them. After reinforcing the teaching plan the nurse ends the visit and schedules a follow-up appointment for the next day to bring written information about two of the medications that the client is taking.

Upon leaving the home, the nurse drives to a nearby shopping center and calls the supervisor at the agency to describe his observations and ask for guidance. The nurse also documents the observations in the client's medical record and completes an incident report. From the description of the situation above, what are the safety issues? Whose safety is of concern to the nurse? What would you tell the supervisor? What type(s) of risk(s) are you dealing with here?

Distasio (2000a, 2000b) argues that home health agencies need a comprehensive violence prevention program to provide staff with necessary strategies to recognize and respond to potentially violent situations. Today, the caseload of many agencies includes clients with behavioral health problems who need counseling and medication management. The nurse in the scenario recognized cues indicative of the pre-assaultive stage. Not just that, the nurse also saw evidence of recent assault(s) and followed the agency's violence prevention protocol. He recognized intuitively that the behavior of the client and his wife was inappropriate and that there was need for additional intervention. Scheduling an appointment for the next day provides an opportunity to gain entry and to explore options for the wife and the client (Christopher & Beck, 1997).

Because threats to safety may come at any place and at any time, community vigilance is required. If a nurse notices an increase in gang presence in a neighborhood or people "hanging out" in front of the client's home, the nursing supervisor should be informed. Has your car been vandalized in the parking lot of an apartment building? Did you have the feeling that you were being watched, or followed when you left the client's home? What evasive action did you take?

Summary

Home visiting is an important nursing intervention that enables clients to obtain continuity of care to manage their health after discharge from the hospital or other health care facility. Nurses may encounter situations that threaten the safety of the client, the agency, and themselves. These threats may occur during each phase of the home visit—the antecedent phase, getting to the home, making the home visit, and leaving the home and returning to the agency.

Factors related to the environment or geographics of the visit, the client, the nurse, and the agency influence the management of threats to safety. Nurses bring personal attributes, beliefs, values, and intuitions to the home visiting situation that enable them to understand the threats and respond to them with available resources. Threats to safety are everywhere; however, the essential factor is the nurses' ability to recognize the situation as threatening and to respond effectively.

OSHA recommends that employers develop policies and guidelines to protect workers from "hazards." The ANA *Code for Nurses* for safety posits that nurses should protect themselves and the client from harm. Assuring safety in home care requires collaboration among all stakeholders. Research has shown that when nurses participate with their agency in designing safety programs that address risk in the workplace and participate in in-service education on the topic, they feel empowered, and are more willing to report experiencing threats to safety and manage them more effectively. In addition, nurses feel supported by their employer. Home care nurses are ultimately responsible for their own safety during the home visit. The environment provides environmental props that can be used to enhance safety. When nurses protect themselves by using observation skills, by trusting their intuitive sense that something is wrong, and by responding in the best interest for themselves and their clients, they are providing a framework for assuring safety.

References

Allender, J. A., & Spradley, B. W. (2005). *Community health nursing: Promoting and protecting the public's health.* Philadelphia: Lippincott Williams & Wilkins.

American Nurses Association. (2001). Retrieved June 15, 2004, from
http://nursingworld.org

Antonovsky, A. (1979). *Health, stress and coping*. San Francisco: Jossey-Bass.

Antonovsky, A. (1984). *Unraveling the mystery of health: How people manage stress and stay well*. San Francisco: Jossey-Bass.

Beech, B. (2001). Sign of the times or the shape of things to come? A 3-day unit of instruction on "aggression and violence in health settings for all students during pre-registration nursing training." *Accident and Emergency Nursing, 9*, 204–211.

Byrd, M. (1995). A concept analysis of home visiting. *Public Health Nursing, 12*(2), 83–89.

Castelli, P., Hart, L. A., & Zasloff, R. L. (2001). Companion cats and the social support systems of men with AIDS. *Psychology Reports, 89*(1), 177–187.

Christopher, M. A., & Beck, T. L. (1997). Caregiver safety. *Journal of Long-Term Care, 16*(1), 32–41.

Denton, M. A., Zeytinoğhu, I. U., & Davies, S. (2002). Working in clients' homes: The impact on the mental health and wellbeing of visiting home care workers. *Home Health Care Services Quarterly, 21*(1), 1-27.

Distasio, C. (2000a). Violence against home care providers: Stop it before it starts. *Caring Magazine, 19*(10), 14-18.

Distasio, C. (2000b, November 27). Planning helps home care RNs stop violence before it starts. *Nursing Spectrum, Career Fitness Online.* Retrieved January 22, 2003, from http://www.community.nursingspectrum.com/MagazineArticles/articles.cfm/AID=2787

Ellenbecker, C. H., Frazier, S. C., & Verney, S. (2004). Nurses' observations and experiences of problems and adverse effects of medication management at home. *Geriatric Nursing, 25*(3), 164-170.

Fazzone, P. A., Barloon, L. F., McConnell, S. J., & Chitty, J. A. (2000). Personal safety, violence and home health. *Public Health Nursing, 17*(1), 43-52.

Feldman, P. H., Sapienza, A. M., & Kane, N. M. (1990). *Who cares for them? Workers in the home care industry.* New York: Greenwood Press.

Gellner, P., Landers, S., O'Rouke, D., & Schlegel, M. (1994). Community health nursing in the 1990s—risky business. *Holistic Nursing Practice, 13*, 90-96.

Jennings, L. B. (1997). Potential benefits of pet ownership in health promotion. *Journal of Holistic Nursing, 15*(4), 358-372.

Kalish, P. A., & Kalish, B. J. (1978). The advance of American nursing. Boston: Little, Brown.

Kendra, M. A., (1996). Perception of risk by home health care administrators and field workers. *Public Health Nursing, 13*(6), 386-393. Erratum: *Public Health Nursing, 14*(6), 401.

Kendra, M. A., & George, V. D. (2001). Defining risk in home visiting. *Public Health Nursing, 18*(2), 128-139.

Kendra, M. A., Weiker, A., Grant, A., Simon, S., & Shullick, D. (1996). Safety concerns affecting delivery of home health care. *Public Health Nursing, 13*(2), 83-87.

Lazarus, R. S. (1966). *Emotion and adaptation.* New York: Oxford University Press.

Lazarus, R. S. (1991). *Psychological stress and coping process.* New York: McGraw-Hill.

Lazarus, R. S., & Folkman, S. (1984). *Stress, appraisal and coping.* New York: Springer.

McPhaul, K. M., & Lipscomb, J. (2004). Workplace violence in health care: Recognized but not regulated. *Online Journal of Issues in Nursing, 9*(3), Manuscript 6. Available: http://www.nursingworld.org/ojin/topic25/tpc25_6.htm

Miller, C. A. (2004). *Nursing for wellness in older adults: Theory and practice* (4th ed.). Philadelphia: Lippincott Williams & Wilkins.

Morris, R., Krueger, C., & Yaross, D. (2004). Better safe than sorry. *Home Healthcare Nurse 22*(6), 417-422.

Paterson, B., McCornish, A., & Bradley, P. (1999). Violence at work. *Nursing Standard, 13*(21), 43-46.

Rowe, W. D. (1977). *An anatomy of risk*. New York: Wiley & Sons.

Sable, P. (1995). Pets, attachment, and well-being across the life cycle. *Social Work, 40*(3), 334-341.

Sitzman, K. (2001). Avoiding random acts of violence. *Home Healthcare Nurse 19*(7), 426-431.

Steinberg, A. (1994). Safety and home care nurses: A study. *Saskatchewan Registered Nurses' Association, 24*(5), 24-26.

Sylvester, B. J., & Reisener, L. (2002). Scared to go to work: A home care performance improvement initiative. *Journal of Nursing Care Quality, 17*(1), 71-82.

U. S. Department of Health and Human Services, Public Health Service, Centers for Disease Control and Prevention, National Institute for Occupational Safety and Health, Division of Safety Research. (1996). *Violence in the workplace. Risk factors and prevention strategies*. Washington, DC: DHHS (NIOSH) Publication No. 96-100. Retrieved July 9, 2004, from http://www.cdc.gov/niosh/violrisk.html)

U. S. Department of Labor, Bureau of Labor Statistics. (2001). *Survey of occupational injuries and illnesses, 2000*. Available: http://www.bls.gov/iif/oshwc/osh/os/osnmr0013.pdf

U. S. Department of Labor, Bureau of Labor Statistics, National Industry-Occupational Employment Matrix, data for 2004. (2004). Retrieved June 23, 2004, from http://www.bls.gov/

U. S. Department of Labor, Occupational Safety and Health Administration. (2004). *Guidelines for preventing workplace violence for health care and social service workers*. (Public Law 91-596, December 29, 1970). OSHA 3148-01R. Retrieved July 15, 2004, from http://www.osha.gov

Chapter 6

Infusion Therapy: High-Tech Home Care Concerns and Issues

Jo Johns, RN, OCN, CRNI

Key Terms

Access Device	Infusion Therapy	Total Parenteral Nutrition (TPN)

The last 10 to 15 years have seen radical changes and increasingly widespread acceptance of home care **infusion therapy,** which is broadly defined as the administration of fluids or medications into the body through the intravenous, subcutaneous, or epidural routes. Insurance companies by challenging the accepted norms, have been a major force in driving the shift of what can acceptably be done in the home setting. But while reimbursement issues may attempt to dictate what can be done in the home setting, it is the responsibility of the home care nurse, along with all members of the health care team, to make informed decisions regarding the safety of the client based on safe nursing practice, agency policy and procedure, and appropriate information regarding the client and the therapy.

Whether in the hospital, outclient, or home setting, the liability of the nurse is basically the same. There must be a physician order for appropriate medication and dosage, and the medication must be administered correctly to the correct client. In addition, in the home setting the client and/or caregiver must have the education needed to administer and store the medication safely as well as care for the **access device.** The access device, sometimes referred to as an access port, is the mechanism by which fluids are infused through the venous system into the body.

Infusion regimes that can be delivered at home include therapies for hydration, chemotherapy, antimicrobials, pain management, cardiac management, and delivery of **total parenteral nutrition (TPN).** TPN, sometimes referred to as hyperalimentation, is "the infusion of a solution containing dextrose, amino acids, fats, essential fatty acids, vitamins, and minerals directly into a vein to meet the client's daily nutritional requirements" (DeLaune & Ladner, 2006, p. 1065.)

Nurse competency is of primary importance when administering infusion therapy. The Standard of Nursing Care is legally defined as "providing reasonable, prudent client care as required by the situation. The care delivered by the nurse must comply with what is expected, given the circumstances in which the care is provided" (Alexander & Webster, 2001, p. 50). Other standards of care are provided by agency policies and procedures, including those of state or federal agencies such as the Centers for Disease Control and Prevention (CDC) and published standards of practice of the professional nursing organizations. The Intravenous Nurses Society (INS), the Oncology Nursing Society (ONS), and others help provide a means for evaluation of client care and nursing competency. A home care agency should establish an internal standard of competency evaluation based on these standards and guidelines (Counce, 2004).

See Chapter 8 for a discussion of standards of practice.

Clinician Safeguards

On November 6, 2000, then-President Bill Clinton signed the Needlestick Safety and Prevention Act into law with an April 18, 2001 compliance date. This law, enforced through the Occupational Safety and Health Administration (OSHA) Division of the U.S. Department of Labor (USDL), was a revised standard of the 1991 Bloodborne Pathogens Standard put in place to protect health care workers from the risk of exposure to bloodborne pathogens (OSHA, 2003). This revised standard clarifies the need for employers to:

- Select and provide safer needle devices.
- Involve employees in identifying and choosing these devices.
- Maintain a log of injuries from contaminated sharps.
- Have a mandatory employee hepatitis B vaccine declination signed if the employee chooses not to receive the hepatitis B vaccine.
  (OSHA, 2003.)

To furnish information regarding blood-borne pathogens and needlestick injuries, OSHA's Office of Occupational Health Nursing (OOHN), OSHA's Office of Occupational Medicine (OOM), and the American Biological Safety Association (ABSA) formed an alliance. This alliance, which can be contacted via the U.S. Department of Labor, helps provide current information and useful tips to assure an optimally safe working environment even when that environment is the client's home (OSHA, 2003).

Setting Priorities

Traditionally, home care has been a service largely established for the elderly client population. As health care costs have escalated, this paradigm is shifting, especially in the area of infusion therapy. For example, it is much less expensive to treat an adolescent requiring six weeks of antibiotic therapy in the home rather than as an inclient in the hospital. In addition, it can also be psychologically beneficial for clients to be in their own home environment during therapy.

A primary concern, before a referral for an infusion therapy client is accepted, is the issue of cost reimbursement. Ethical concerns are raised when a client receives a therapy for which he or she assumed Medicare or insurance would be financially responsible, when in reality that is not the case. It is imperative that clients know what costs will be personally incurred prior to receiving infusion therapy in the home or any other setting.

Medicare has strict and restrictive guidelines regarding which infusion therapies are reimbursable, frequently making infusion therapy in the home setting cost-prohibitive for a client with Medicare-only reimbursement. Medicare supplemental insurance helps pay for the 20% that Medicare does not pay on Medicare-approved therapies. A Medicare secondary insurance will usually help pay for therapies that are not Medicare-reimbursable (Fetter, 2003; Fitzpatrick, 1999). Medicaid reimbursement for infusion therapies varies by state and type of therapy. Therapy reimbursement can also vary between a child and an adult. There can even be state-to-state variances of the ages that constitute adulthood (Fitzpatrick, 1999).

Private insurance companies employ case managers who help establish the reimbursement guidelines for clients requiring home infusion. Minimally, the issues addressed include the cost(s) of (1) medication, diluent, and fees incurred with medication preparation; (2) pump rental; (3) ancillary supplies; (4) costs for which the client is responsible such as deductibles; and (5) issues related to frequency and necessity of home care visits (Fitzpatrick, 1999).

It is imperative that the nurses (always Registered Nurses) who are in communication with the case managers are knowledgeable about the client status, disease process, access device, therapy administration, medication, its possible untoward effects, and administration device. The availability of the home care nurse to the client will hinge on the case management of the client's individual situation. The client, case manager, and health care provider must realize that home health care is intermittent care, not private duty, and that the client and/or caregiver will have to be able to assume responsibility for the bulk of the care. The most important consideration when arranging home infusion therapy should always be client safety.

Client Assessment for Home Infusion Therapy

Assessment of the potential client for home infusion therapy is not always possible, other than through dialogue with the health care provider or referral person. There are many questions that must be addressed to provide the safest setting, individualized therapy, and access device for the client. General areas of concern and sample assessment questions will now be discussed.

Condition of the Client and the Environment   The assessment of any client in home care begins with the client and includes both the client's home environment and the client's caregivers (Fitzpatrick, 1999). Sample assessment questions include:

- What is the physical condition of the client?
- What is the client's age?
- What are the physical and emotional limitations of the client?

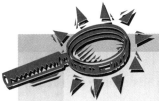

Evidence-Based Practice Box 6-1

Success in Teaching Infusion Therapy to Family Caregivers

Many factors have influenced the need for family caregivers to administer infusion therapy in the home. This is often an anxiety-producing event, especially when most of these caregivers are facing life-threatening diagnoses of their loved ones.

A grounded research study by Cox and Westbrook (2005) investigated caregivers' feelings about learning home infusion therapy. Themes ranged from "Can I do this?" to "What was helpful and not helpful in my learning?"

Using the caregivers' input, the researchers were able to identify tips for nurses when teaching home infusion therapy. Tips included simplifying the training; explaining all of the steps, even the small ones; understanding the anxiety; and keeping the teaching relaxed and low-key, not drastic or melodramatic. (See page 104 of Cox and Westbrook for the complete list of tips.) Additionally, guidelines for a successful infusion therapy educational process were established (see Cox and Westbrook page 106).

This research study suggests that developing competence in home caregivers' infusion skills is related to nurses' own teaching skills. The study offers helpful information for the nurses to reach that goal.

- What are the pertinent diagnoses of the client?
- What is the height and weight of the client?
- Does the client have any allergies and, if so, what type and severity of reaction occurs?
- Is the client able to assist in therapy administration?
- Are the client and family educable regarding the therapy, infection control, possible adverse events, and equipment management?
- Is there someone willing to assume care if the client is not able?
- Who is that person?
- Is this home setting an appropriate environment for the therapy ordered?

Some clinicians recommend that, once home care infusion clients become 65 years of age, a geriatric assessment is in order. Typically a geriatric assessment is "a multidimensional, diagnostic process used to establish medical, psychosocial, and functional status and problems, and develop an overall plan for care and follow-up" (Fetter, 2003, p. 155).

Therapy Administration   After completion of the client and home assessment, the nurse proceeds to assessment and data collection related to the client's therapy. Questions in this area include:

- What is the therapy?
- What is the anticipated length of the therapy?

- What type of access device does the client have (or need)?
- Can the maintenance and care be based on agency policy?
- If there are variances, what are they?
- What is the frequency of the therapy?
- What are the administration times of the therapy and can the times be adjusted if necessary?
- When is the last dose prior to coming home?
- When is the next dose due?
- What pertinent laboratory values are needed and how often are they to be drawn?
- What are the client's laboratory values prior to coming home (especially abnormal values)?

Health Care Provider   The health care provider delivering infusion therapy to home care clients will be a registered nurse (RN). The RN should, through experience, be an infusion therapy expert, or may be certified in infusion therapy. The nurse not only delivers the infusion therapy but also provides emotional support, encouragement, and consultation to the client and caregiver who are often frightened by the therapy. Questions to be considered are:

- What are the services being allowed by the payor?
- Who are the primary health care providers and what are the contact numbers, including fax numbers and pager numbers?
- What are the laboratory abnormalities?
- Are there any specific changes in the client's status?

It is necessary that there be good communication between all members of the health care team to establish the safest care possible. This is especially true between the infusion company and the home care agency.

Infusion Access Devices

There are several types of access devices available to home care infusion clients. All infusion devices are invasive and require competent, diligent care. Following is a list, with definitions, of the access devices most frequently used in home care.

- Subcutaneous infusion (SQ) device: an access needle with cannula inserted and stabilized into the subcutaneous tissue.
- Peripheral intravenous access (PIV) device: a short catheter used to access peripheral veins.
- Central venous access device (CVAD): a long catheter that is threaded through the venous system until it reaches the superior vena cava.

Careful consideration of the type of access device implanted into a client is important, but decisions are not always based on what is the best access device for this therapy, this client, and in this home setting especially when compared to the inclient setting. Some considerations that should have bearing when the choice of access device is made minimally include:

1. What is the diagnosis of the client? There is a great deal of difference between a cancer client undergoing chemotherapy and someone requiring only several days of hydration therapy.

2. What is the anticipated length of therapy? Is this a six-week course of antibiotics or a six-month session of bowel rest with the necessity of total parenteral nutrition?
3. What reimbursement is available? Is the access device the most cost effective?
4. What is the best choice for the abilities and limitations of the client and/or caregiver?
5. What are the properties of the medication or infusion? Is this a hyperosmolar, extreme pH or vesicant (caustic) solution that requires administration through a central venous access device (CVAD), or an isotonic solution for three days of hydration?

Flushing an intravenous access device, peripheral or central, is based on the "SASH" method, which is:

Saline→ Administration of medication→ Saline→ Heparin

The rationale for this method is based on the fact that although heparin is used to help maintain intravenous access patency, there are many medication incompatibilities that can occur with heparin. Figure 6-1 demonstrates the SASH procedure.

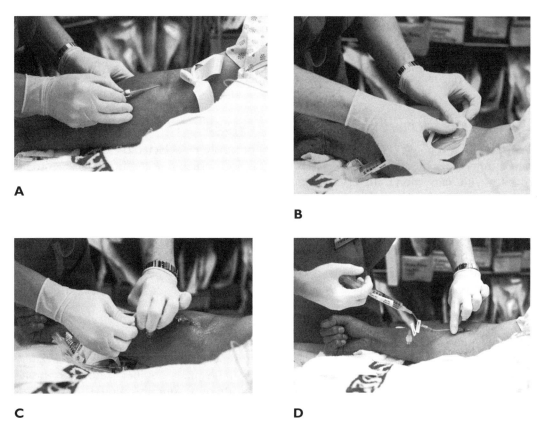

A

B

C   **D**

Figure 6-1 The SASH method for flushing an IV access device. **A.** Insert an over-the-needle catheter. **B.** Cover the site with a transparent dressing. **C.** Screw the heparin lock onto the hub of the extension tubing. **D.** Inject saline slowly into the lock and extension tubing.

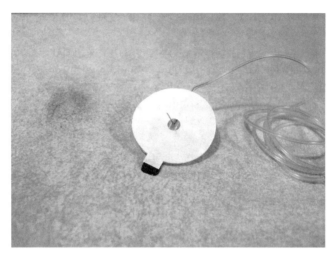

Figure 6-2 Subcutaneous infusion set.

Subcutaneous Infusion Devices

Subcutaneous (SQ) infusion may be indicated for some continuous therapies. In SQ infusion therapy, the access device is a needle with attached cannula that is inserted into the subcutaneous tissue (Figure 6-2). The site, which is easily accessed by the client or caregiver, is usually rotated every five to seven days (Gorski & Czaplewski, 1999).

Peripheral Intravenous Access Devices

Peripheral intravenous (PIV) access devices are appropriate for selected therapies. It is important to remember that in the home setting there is not a nurse outside the client's bedroom to assist with reinsertion if the PIV malfunctions. It is also worth noting that even though the PIV may be a less costly product, it is possible that greater cost may be incurred with infiltration, malfunction, or nursing visits for reinsertion, while limiting client mobility and quality of life. Figure 6-3 shows two types of PIV catheters.

Complications   As with any invasive procedure, the potential for complications arises. Many complications can be prevented or lessened in severity by prevention, early detection, and most especially, good client education about what is reportable.

Central Venous Access Devices

A true central venous access device (CVAD) is an IV catheter that is threaded through the venous system ending several centimeters into the superior vena cava. CVADs are advantageous in many ways for clients who require therapy in hospitals, outclient settings, or home settings, and to the nurses facilitating the care and therapy administration. These devices can increase hemodilution of the infusate, decrease discomfort associated with frequent peripheral venipunctures, decrease missed doses, and diminish potential for infiltration, extravasation, and catheter migration.

Because of the lumen size of CVADs, the pressure per square inch (psi) incurred with the use of a syringe smaller than 10 cc volume is contraindicated. Too much pressure from a

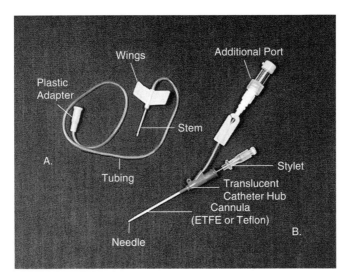

Figure 6-3 Peripheral intravenous access devices.
A. Butterfly **B.** Angiocatheter

smaller syringe could potentially rupture the catheter, resulting in life-threatening consequences for the client.

Infusion therapies that require a CVAD are continuous infusion of vesicant chemotherapy, because of its tissue irritant properties; continuous infusion of the cardiac medications dobutamine and milrinone, because of the dangers associated with therapy interruption; and total parenteral nutrition, because its high glucose and protein content may be tissue-caustic.

It is worth noting that a client receiving TPN alone to meet all of his caloric needs must take some fluid or substance orally or via an enteral tube to maintain a healthy bacterial state of the colon. It is possible, if a client takes nothing by mouth or enterally, for the normal bacteria of the gut to translocate to another site in the body, especially a site where a foreign object resides. A CVAD is a foreign object in the client and can become a receptacle of translocated bacteria, which can result in sepsis. This complication requires antimicrobials and removal of the device. Even sips of water can help prevent this situation.

Peripherally Inserted Central Catheter   A peripherally inserted central catheter (PICC) is a type of CVAD that is inserted through the venous system of an extremity (usually the cephalic or basilic veins) into the subclavian vein and then into the superior vena cava.

Non-Tunneled CVAD   A non-tunneled CVAD is a catheter that is inserted surgically into the chest area and directly threaded into the subclavian vein and then into the superior vena cava. Figure 6-4 shows the tips of CVAD catheters as they reside in the vena cava.

Tunneled CVAD   A tunneled CVAD is a catheter that is surgically inserted, usually in the chest area, through subcutaneous tissue before being inserted into the subclavian vein. It is then threaded into the superior vena cava. Figure 6-5 illustrates a tunneled catheter.

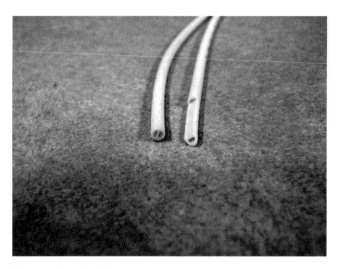

Figure 6-4 CVAD tips, demonstrating the multilumens as they reside in the vena cava.

Implanted CVAD (Implanted Port)   An implanted CVAD is a catheter surgically tunneled into the subcutaneous tissue of the chest or antecubital fossa prior to insertion into the subclavian vein and threaded into the superior vena cava. There is no external catheter, but a port reservoir that is implanted under the skin and then sutured into place and accessed with a non-coring needle (previously called a Huber needle). Figure 6-6 illustrates a side view of a non-coring needle.

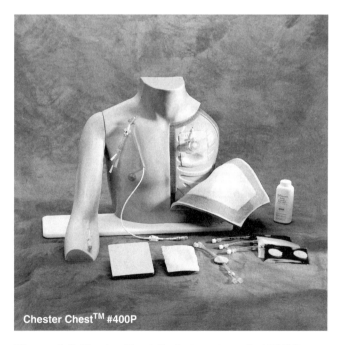

Chester Chest™ #400P

Figure 6-5 Chester Chest illustrates a tunneled CVAD. *(Courtesy VATA Anatomical Health Care Models.)*

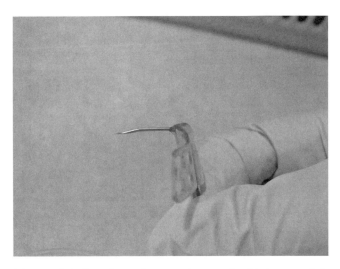

Figure 6-6 Side view of non-coring needle (Huber needle).

Pumps and Infusion Delivery Systems

There are various delivery systems, ranging from the simple to the complex, available for administering infusions. Even the most complex delivery systems are much more user friendly than systems of the past. Manufacturers now realize that the more complex the pump, the less likely it will reassure a client or nurse about its use in the home setting. Careful planning based on the client, the therapy, and the CVAD will help make decisions about the transition home much easier.

Intravenous Push (IV Push) Medications

Intravenous push, also known as direct injection, "is the administration of a drug directly into the venous access device or through the injection port of a continuous infusion set" (Douglas & Hedrick, 2001, p. 182). IV push medications, because of the possibility of damage to delicate venous tissue, are not appropriate for all types of IV therapies. Some of the types of therapies that are appropriate for IV push are those medications or infusions that are minimally caustic to veins and those medications that can be safely administered without danger to cardiac or renal function.

Administration of IV push medications requires equipment that is unique to this type of therapy. For an occasional infusion, a butterfly (steel-winged catheter) (Figure 6-7) or over-the-needle type is adequate. A peripherally inserted central catheter (PICC) is indicated when therapy is expected to be longer than one to two weeks, when a client's venous status is poor, or if medication prepared with consideration of stability and compatibility has the potential for irritation.

Administration of medications via IV push offers advantages such as minimal cost, ease of administration, and minimal client/caregiver education. Additionally, pediatric infusions may benefit from shorter time restriction with decreased restlessness for the child.

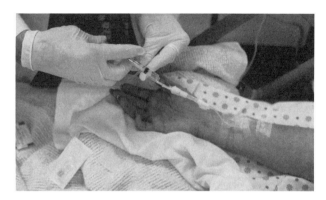

Figure 6-7 IV push using butterfly.

As with all medication therapies there are issues of concern. With administration of IV push medications, the issues are possibly frequent replacement of PIV, concerns about the rate of infusion depending on the infusion or medication, and the increased risk of chemical phlebitis.

Medication Delivery via Gravity or Dial-a-Flow Pumps

Delivery of IV medications by gravity or by a predetermined drop rate is familiar to most people and remains the delivery choice for many infusion therapies. Some infusion therapies are not appropriate for administration by IV push because the medication, when delivered quickly, is tissue-caustic. Delivery by gravity or dial-a-flow is appropriate for medications that require more than usual hydration and/or increased time for safe administration.

Venous access is dependent on client status, frequency of infusion, and length of therapy. An adjustable IV pole offers cost containment, ease of administration, and less education. Most people know what an IV or "drip" is.

Potential for too rapid or too slow an infusion time is always an issue of concern with infusion therapy. Because client position may affect delivery rate, it is recommended that with the use of a dial-a-flow, the infusate container be 36 inches above heart level. When a PICC is the infusion device, the rate of delivery may depend on the lumen size of a PICC. For all types of delivery systems, diligence by the nurse is expected.

Stationary (Pole-Mounted) Pumps

Medications that require structured infusion administration time, nocturnal TPN infusion, hydration of short duration, administration of blood products, and intermittent therapies are especially suited to a pole-mounted pump. The stability of the venous access device—which is dependent on client status, frequency of infusion, and length of therapy—is a consideration for use of the pole-mounted pump. A pole-mounted pump is advantageous when the infusate volume is large, as this method can offer some physical support of infusate bags. This delivery method also offers a pressure per square inch that can maintain timely, effective infusion time with a narrow-lumen PICC.

The issues of concern with this type of pump are (1) the pole and pump may be difficult to push, especially around carpet, furniture, and the bathroom; (2) it could overturn, so it must be used cautiously with children; (3) the internal battery must be charged using an electrical outlet, which brings forward the issue of the length of time that back up power will last in the event of a power outage; and (4) the prevention of free flow should the tubing come loose from pump.

Elastomeric Pumps

An elastomeric pump is a plastic, disposable device that contains a balloon-like inner chamber that, when filled with infusate, will infuse at a specific rate when unclamped. This pump is appropriate for use with intermittent infusions of medications and/or solutions. The pump requires a stable venous access device, which is, as always, dependent on client status, frequency of infusion, and length of therapy.

The advantages of this pump are that it (1) is small and easy to use, (2) has enough pressure per square inch to accommodate a PICC access device, (3) is frequently cost effective, (4) is disposable, (5) is easily handled by children and the elderly, (6) is not dependent on gravity, and (7) requires minimal client education.

The disadvantages of the elastomeric pump are few; however, the pump needs to be primed, raising a potential problem if the infusion dosage needs to be adjusted; and its small size may make it difficult for the elderly to manipulate.

Ambulatory Pumps

An ambulatory infusion pump is about the size of a paperback book. It can be worn around the waist or over the shoulder in a carrying case. This infusion pump is appropriate for continuous infusions, for pain management, and for intermittent infusions of medications that are stable at room temperature for various lengths of time.

The pump requires batteries, a carrying case, a bolus cord for pain management that includes a prescription for as-needed dosing, a stable access device for intravenous or intraspinal infusions, and pump-specific tubing. The advantages of this pump are (1) that gravity is not a concern; (2) ease of use; (3) availability of multiple programmed delivery modes, such as intermittent therapies with keep vein open (KVO) rate between doses, or pain-management therapy (bolus only, bolus + continuous, or continuous without bolus); (4) the therapy program can be locked internally into the pump to prevent manipulation; and (5) the client is usually grateful for the compactness of this ambulatory pump.

Issues of concern for the ambulatory pump include (1) increased cost of a more complicated pump and pump-specific tubing and equipment; (2) the priming volume must be taken into consideration when programming the pump; (3) prevention of free flow is imperative; (4) the time of new container change should be scheduled at times when the client/caregiver would be awake and available; (5) there must be adequate infusate in the home to ensure that uninterrupted therapies are safely maintained; (6) the infusate containers should be changed at times that are best for the client's lifestyle; and (7) there is a need for increased client/caregiver education including pump training as well as training with associated equipment and the therapy itself.

Intraspinal Infusions

Intraspinal catheters are of two types: (1) epidural catheters, which are inserted into the epidural space; and (2) intrathecal catheters, which are inserted into the intrathecal space. In the home setting, these catheters can be used for the administration of antineoplastic chemotherapy or for the administration of pain management medications (Ferrini & Paice, 2004). The equipment needed for intraspinal catheters is specific to the catheter and therapy itself. These catheters, not unlike CVADs, can be external tunneled catheters, implanted ports, implanted pumps, or temporary catheters.

Although there are serious concerns related to intraspinal infusion therapy, these catheters can be an effective way to treat central nervous system neoplasms or various types of pain. Because of the potential for infection and its consequences to the brain and spinal cord, infection control and thorough client/caregiver education is extremely important. Many times these catheters are accessed in an outclient setting but the home care nurse manages the client at home. It becomes the nurse's responsibility to identify signs of catheter/pump malfunction and to educate the client/caregiver in these signs and the interventions appropriate to the problems. Pain infusions must be carefully calculated, because the epidural dose of morphine sulfate is only 1/10th of the intravenous dose. Intrathecal dosing is only 1/100th of the intravenous dose of morphine sulfate.

It remains to be seen if there will be an increase in intraspinal therapies in the home setting, but the case management of the client's care remains the primary concern of the home care nurse. Note that recommendations from the individual state boards of nursing can differ widely on what is acceptable practice in the home setting with regard to clients requiring intraspinal therapies (Perucca, 2001).

Infusion Adapters and Caps

With the increased risk of blood-borne pathogens, fewer needles and needle insertion devices are acceptable for use in any client care setting. There are many infusion adapters and caps that are used as part of needle-protected or needleless systems that help create a safe environment for health care providers and clients. Some adapters even have the added benefit of a positive pressure capacity. That is to say, that when a catheter with an attached adapter is flushed, a positive pressure valve prevents blood particles from being drawn back into the device. Blood particle accumulation can potentially result in blood clot occlusion of the CVAD and provides an optimal opportunity for microbial growth.

A second function of infusion adapters is to maintain a closed system. A closed system helps prevent the instillation of microbes into the body, and even more importantly, helps to prevent the occurrence of air emboli or bleeding from the client. Minimal infusion adapter changes should be performed weekly, whenever blood has been in the cap as in the case of obtaining a blood sampling, and whenever the adapter's sterility has been compromised.

Client and Caregiver Education

Client education is a process, a work in progress based on the client's needs and abilities. Through careful assessment of the client's abilities and knowledge base, goals are set and the process proceeds as the plan of care. The plan of care requires frequent reassessment and evaluation for effectiveness. The information must also be presented with understanding of the client/caregiver abilities or limitations.

Client education should also include return demonstration of techniques that have been taught. The client and supporting caregiver should understand what variables should be recorded or reported and in what manner. The various roles of all involved parties should be defined (who does what), and any education performed necessitates evaluation of understanding and effectiveness. Written communication should be reviewed and left in the home when possible.

Client/caregiver education must minimally include:

- Medication concerns
  - Anticipated side effects.
  - Possible untoward reportable side effects.
  - Medication incompatibilities.
  - Delayed or missed doses.
  - Checks for precipitates and expiration dates.
  - Adequate necessary supplies.
  - Assurance of adequate medication and equipment until the next delivery.
  - Knowledge of requirements for refrigeration and temperature range.
- Infection control issues
  - Good hand-washing.
  - When in doubt—throw it out.
  - Aseptic technique and safe storage of medication and equipment.
  - Frequent/regular body temperature check, and cleanliness of the home setting, especially storage areas.
- Storage and disposable concerns
  - Childproof.
  - Temperature-safe.
  - Correct use of needle-disposal containers.
  - Knowledge related to expired or contaminated medication.
- Client/caregiver knowledge related to access device
  - Signs and symptoms of device malfunction
    - Redness.
    - Pain.
    - Hardness at site.
    - Leakage at the insertion site.
    - Signs of catheter migration.
    - Signs and symptoms of infection.
- Client/caregiver knowledge related to pump
  - Start/stop, battery change, or recharge of pump.
  - Identify malfunction and appropriate interventions.
  - Location and availability of emergency services.
  - Emergency numbers and contacts.
  - How and when to report an unusual finding or circumstance.

Summary

Infusion therapy in the home can be done safely and cost-effectively with appropriate planning and team sharing. Ultimately, decisions should be based on what is best for the client. There remain therapies that are more safely done in the inclient or outclient facility. These decisions can be achieved by carefully planning and assessing the individual issues and needs of each client circumstance, reviewing Nurse Practice Acts of the geographical location, and familiarizing oneself with the State Board of Nursing recommendations. There can be successful client outcomes when agency responsibility and accountability for establishing competency requirements are present. This means that staff training includes federal law mandates for the safety of the client and the health care provider.

References

Alexander, M. C., & Webster, H. K. (2001). Legal aspects of intravenous nursing. In J. Hawkins, R. A. W. Lonsway, C. Hedrick, & M. B. Perdue (Eds.), *Infusion therapy in clinical practice* (2nd ed., pp. 50–64). St. Louis: Saunders.

Counce, J. (2004). Cultivating nursing competencies. *Infusion, 10*(1),12–18.

Cox, J., & Westbrook, L. J. O. (2005). Home infusion therapy: Essential characteristics of a successful education process. A grounded study. *Journal of Infusion Nursing, 28*(2), 99–107.

DeLaune, S. E., & Ladner, P. K. (2006). *Fundamentals of nursing: Standards & practice* (3rd ed.). Clifton Park, NY: Thomson Delmar Learning.

Douglas, J. B., & Hedrick, C. (2001). Pharmacology. In J. Hawkins, R. A. W. Lonsway, C. Hedrick, & M. B. Perdue, (Eds.), *Infusion therapy in clinical practice* (2nd ed., pp. 176–208). St. Louis: Saunders.

Ferrini, R., & Paice, J. A. (2004). How to initiate and monitor infusional lidocaine for severe and/or neuropathic pain. *Journal of Supportive Oncology, 2*(1), 90–94.

Fetter, M. S. (2003). Geriatric assessment and management protocols: Issues for home infusion therapy providers. *Journal of Infusion Nursing, 26*(3), 153–160.

Fitzpatrick, L. M. (1999). Care and management issues regarding central venous access devices in the home and long-term care setting. *Journal of Intravenous Nursing, 22*(6S), S40–S45.

Gorski, L.A., & Czaplewski, L. M. (1999). Basic concepts in infusion therapy. In L.A. Gorski (Ed.) *Best practices in home infusion therapy* (pp. 7:1–7:64). Gaithersburg, MD: Aspen.

Occupational Safety and Health Administration, U. S. Department of Labor. (2003). *Safety and health topics: Bloodborne pathogens and needlestick prevention.* Retrieved June 25, 2004, from
http://www.osha-slc.gov/SLTC/bloodbornepathogens/index.html

Perucca, R. (2001). Infusion therapy equipment. In J. Hawkins, R. A. W. Lonsway, C. Hedrick, & M. B. Perdue (Eds.), *Infusion therapy in clinical practice* (2nd ed., pp. 300–333). St. Louis: Saunders.

Part II

Administrative Operations

Chapter 7

Leadership

Andrea McCall, RN, BSN

Key Terms

Governing Body	Leadership Team	Scope of Services

The **leadership team** in a home care agency is responsible for providing the overall direction for the agency. The leadership team's responsibilities include business planning, budgeting, human resource planning, emergency management, performance improvement, and customer relations. The leadership team has a clear background understanding of the agency's corporate status, financial designation, mission, goals, and objectives. Although each of these items will influence the overall planning and operational policies of an agency, client care decisions are ultimately made on the basis of the needs of clients independent of finances.

A home care agency may or may not be certified by the Centers for Medicare and Medicaid Services (CMS). Medicare certification is necessary to provide home care services to Medicare beneficiaries and Medicaid recipients. Non-Medicare certified agencies may not provide visiting services to clients who are Medicare or Medicaid beneficiaries. Other examples of home care services include private duty care, in-home aide services, durable medical equipment, and home infusion pharmacy services. An agency may provide one, all, or any combination of these services depending upon licensure laws and regulations governing the provision of home care services in its state and the scope of services defined by the agency's governing body. For purposes of the leadership and management responsibilities discussed in this chapter, the assumption will be made that the home care agency is Medicare certified.

Home care agencies are designated as for-profit or not-for-profit; this will influence the agency leadership's direction and decision-making. A for-profit agency, which looks to its leaders to provide a yearly profit, may be a privately owned company with an individual or a group of owners, or a publicly owned company traded on a stock exchange responsible to its shareholders for its performance. Shareholders expect the agency to provide a positive return on their financial investment in the agency either through growth in the value and therefore price of the agency, or through sharing of profits in the form of dividends. The leadership team must balance the operational needs of the agency and its clients with the financial performance expectations of its owners when making its decisions.

In addition to understanding the agency's financial status, the leadership team understands the agency's operational status, which may be hospital based, free-standing, or part of a multi-office entity. This status may influence the planning and operational decisions of the leadership team. For example, the primary mission and goal of a hospital-based agency may be to provide support to its hospital. Support may be achieved through the development of programs that assist the hospital in its efforts to lower hospital in-client length of stay, lowering the hospital census, and providing a continuum of care from the hospital while serving the residents of the community. On the other hand, a non–hospital-based agency may choose to develop relationships with several hospitals, physicians, and others in the community with a goal of providing care to as many clients as possible while meeting its financial goals. A community based nonprofit agency may exist to serve the home care needs of its community with financial goals obtained through a combination of billing revenue, fund raising, grants, and public funds.

Governance

Regardless of financial status, ownership, or affiliation, each agency has a **governing body,** which has the ultimate legal authority and responsibility for the overall operation of the agency. The Medicare Conditions of Participations for Home Health Agencies Standard 484.14(b) states that "a governing body (or designated persons so functioning) assumes full legal authority and responsibility for the operation of the agency." The governing body establishes the mission, vision, and goals of the home care agency. Operationally, the governing body is responsible for the home care agency budget, **scope of services** (types of services) to be provided, approval of policies and procedures, and the appointment of the agency administrator. The governing body also conducts an annual evaluation of the services provided by the home care agency. When the home care agency is part of a larger organization such as a hospital or multi-branch organization, regardless of whether the facility is a nonprofit or for-profit, the governing body may review and provide approval of the actions presented by the home care agency administrator on behalf of the leadership team (CMS, 2004a).

Advisory Group

The governing body appoints an advisory group, which is made up of professional personnel who represent the scope of services provided by the home care agency. Members of the group include a physician and a nurse, at least one of whom is not employed by the agency, and consumers from the community that the home care agency serves. The members of the advisory group provide input and insight to assist the agency in its development, provision of programs, and services for the community. Annually, the advisory group conducts the agency program evaluation and presents its findings and recommendations to the governing body.

The Leadership Team

The leadership team is further defined within the agency. Depending upon the size and type of the agency, the governing body and the leadership team may be one and the same, a blend of governing body members and management team members of the agency, or separate entities with no overlap in membership. For example, in a large multi-branch or hospital-based agency, the leadership team responsible for the daily operational decisions and the governing body may be separate entities, with the leadership team having a reporting relationship to the governing body.

Each agency defines its leadership team. Although the team may or may not be defined in writing, the members of the leadership team should be visibly evident in the home care agency. The leadership team may consist of as few or as many members as the agency deems necessary depending upon its status (discussed above) and its management philosophy. Agency leadership may consist of a team as small as the administrator, clinical director, and financial director. At the other end of the spectrum, an agency may define its leadership team so that it consists of the administrator and management personnel from the departments of clinical services, finance, information services, marketing, community relations, and quality/performance improvement. The agency may further limit its defined leadership as the head of each of these areas or may also include lower level management staff. Regardless of the size or position components of the team, its functions and responsibilities within the agency are the same.

Home Care Administrator   The governing body appoints the home health administrator, who is responsible for the daily operations of the home care agency. This position, which is required in a Medicare-certified home care agency, may be held by a licensed physician, registered nurse, or a person who has training and experience in health service administration and at least one year of supervisory experience in home health care or related health programs (CMS, 2004b).

The administrator is responsible for assuring that the home care agency is compliant with all required laws and regulations. If an accrediting body such as the Joint Commission (JC) or the Community Health Accreditation Program (CHAP) also accredits the home care agency, the administrator must assure that the agency complies with the accrediting organization's standards as well. The administrator serves as the liaison between the home care agency leadership team and the governing body. There must be an alternate person, designated in writing, for this position when the administrator is unavailable.

Director of Nurses   When the home care administrator is not a physician or a registered nurse, state laws regulating home care agencies may require a home care agency to appoint a director of nursing (DON). In this case, the director of nursing, sometimes called the director of clinical services, holds a key leadership position. The qualifications for the DON usually include graduation from an accredited school of nursing, unencumbered licensure in the state in which the home care agency provides services, and clinical experience. It is desirable that this nursing leader holds a baccalaureate degree in nursing from a program approved by the National League for Nursing or public health nursing preparation. As with the administrator's position, there must be an alternate designated in writing to act in the absence of the DON (CMS, 2004c).

The DON must be on the premises or available by telecommunications at all times during the operating hours of the agency. The DON is aware of and participates in all activities relevant to the services furnished by the agency. Development of qualifications and the assignment of personnel also are within the scope of the DON's role (CMS, 2004c).

Financial Services Leader   Strong financial management is an essential component of a successful home care agency. Essential qualifications and experience for the financial management leader include a bachelor's degree in a business or accounting-related field, computer skills, and experience in health care related financial services including billing and collections. The key responsibilities of the financial services leader include preparing budgets, billing, and collecting payment for the services provided. The financial services leader also provides the other members of the leadership team with ongoing analysis of financial trends within the agency. Such analysis requires (1) preparation of financial impact projections to assist in the assessment of service lines under consideration or in development, (2) analysis of the potential impact to the agency of contract arrangements, and (3) tracking the costs of providing services to the home care agency's clients. At least annually, the financial services leader will prepare, or in the case of a multi-branch or hospital-based home care agency, participate in the preparation of a cost report. The home care agency cost report is a report of the services provided by the home care agency and the costs of providing the services. The report is prepared and submitted annually to the fiscal intermediary designated by the Centers for Medicare and Medicaid Services.

Information Management Leader   Information management is vital to the success of any health care business. Information management in the home care agency is inclusive of written, spoken, and electronic information. Information management leadership assures the standardization of information, including medical records, and facilitates efficient and effective communications throughout the home care agency. The information management leader participates in the selection of computer programs that meet agency needs, development of management reports, and provision of support systems for staff using the information management systems. The information management leader possesses skills in the areas of computer technology, medical records formatting, electronic documentation, and report development. The information manager must be skilled in all aspects of computer literacy and may hold a degree in Management Information Systems, but such a degree is not necessary.

Performance Improvement and Quality Manager   Performance improvement and quality management is the responsibility of everyone in a home care agency; however, many home care agencies will designate a team member to lead the performance improvement activities of the agency. Performance improvement can be defined as "the study and adaptation of functions and processes to increase the probability of achieving desired outcomes" (JCAHO, 1999, p. 164). The effective leader in this position will possess skills and experience in the areas of teamwork, communication, performance improvement methodology, and statistical analysis. Although a health care background is helpful, in large organizations with multiple staff in quality management positions, a clinical background is not essential for the performance improvement manager to be an effective leader within the home care agency.

Specialty Leadership Positions   Large home care agencies may offer multiple services, each requiring its own group of specialists and therapists and necessitating their own managers. Additional leadership positions that may be present in a home care agency, and their typical qualifications, include the following:

1. Therapy services leader is a registered nurse or licensed therapist with a minimum of one year of experience in home care. His or her primary functions would include supervision of all physical, speech, and occupational therapists and assistants.

2. Clinical supervisory staff members are usually registered nurses with a minimum of one year of experience in home care. They are responsible for the supervision of a group of nursing staff or clients.

3. Home infusion program leader is a physician, registered nurse, registered pharmacist, or other health care executive with a minimum of a bachelor's degree in
   a health care related field or equivalent experience. He or she is responsible for
   the oversight of all infusion services to patients in an outpatient setting.

4. Home medical equipment program leader is a respiratory therapist, registered
   nurse, physician, or other health care manager with a minimum of a bachelor's
   degree in a health care related field. This individual is responsible for the provision and oversight of medical equipment and respiratory services.

5. In-home aide services program leader is a registered nurse with a minimum of one
   year of home care experience. He or she is responsible for the clinical oversight
   and assignment of aide services.

6. Community relations or marketing manager is a health care professional, usually a
   registered nurse, or a person active and well known in the community that the
   agency serves. A background in sales and marketing is helpful. This manager is
   responsible for physician and other health care professionals' education concerning home care services.

Other leadership positions may be developed as necessary depending upon the overall
structure of the home care agency or if a home care agency develops specialty programs as
part of its scope of services. Examples of additional programs that may require the development of additional leadership positions are a dedicated home care pediatrics program or a
telehealth program. Home care agencies that are part of a larger organization may have other
leadership positions within their hospital or corporate structure that will interact with the
home care agency leadership team as needed.

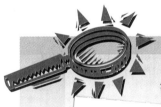

Evidence-Based Practice Box 7-1

g Nursing Leaders for the Future

Tod... erned about the lack of interest shown in leadership posi-
tio... urses. Today's leaders are products of the baby-boom
ge... rs will be products of Generation X. Differences in values
an... generations need to be addressed to establish a pool of
p... future.
... was conducted in south Florida with 48 participants who
w... s. Input was gathered relating to role responsibilities, control
in decision ...... , compensation, and other related topics (Sherman, 2005).

Important results from the study revealed that potential nursing leaders need "mentors,
administrative support, education related to leadership, support of nursing staff, and elimination of barriers to move up into nursing leadership positions" (Sherman, 2005, p. 130).

Also mentioned was the necessity for present nursing leaders to share the positive
aspects of their roles with younger staff.

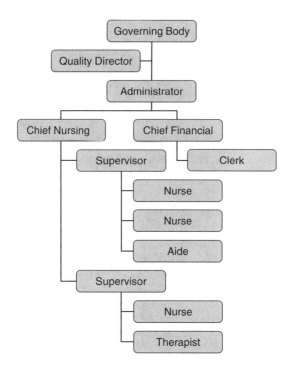

Figure 7-1 Top-down organizational chart with administration at the top.

Organizational Structure

The leadership team defines the operational structure and reporting relationships of the organization under the direction of the governing body. The organizational structure is defined and conveyed to all agency staff through the use of organizational charts.

Organizational Charts

Organizational charts may be structured in a variety of ways. Charts may show functional relationships, may be defined by job titles, or may even give the individual names of staff members. Some organizational charts reflect a "top-down" approach, with the governing body or administrator at the top of the chart and organizational lines demonstrating the flow of authority down throughout the organization (Figure 7-1).

Other organizational charts may start with the client as the top of the chart with all other functions flowing up to support client care. Dotted lines may be used to indicate shared responsibilities or interdepartmental relationships (Figure 7-2). A more unusual organizational

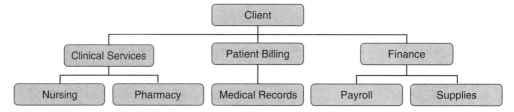

Figure 7-2 Top-down organizational chart with client at the top.

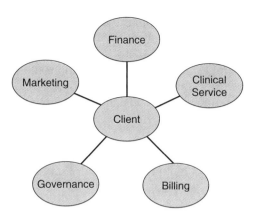

Figure 7-3 Circular organizational chart with client in the center.

chart may be presented in a circular format, with the client at the center of the circle and all other agency functions and personnel shown as circles around the client, demonstrating a concept of client-centered care (Figure 7-3).

Home care agencies that are part of a hospital or large multi-branch organization may have several organizational charts. Additional organizational charts should be developed demonstrating the agency's relationship to its parent organization, governing body, and other related departments or entities.

Policies and Procedures

Policies and procedures are developed to provide guidance to all home care agency staff on how the home care agency expects its staff to provide client care and conduct business. Policies and procedures are developed to provide both administrative and clinical practice guidance to staff. The home care agency leadership team is responsible for developing a process for the development of policies and procedures within the agency and the communication of these policies and procedures to all staff within the home care agency. In developing its policies and procedures, the agency should consider the agency's mission, vision, goals, and scope of services. Additional policy items that are considered as appropriate to the individual agency include applicable laws, regulations, and community or professional standards of care.

Home care agencies that are accredited by an accrediting body must also assure that the agency's policies and procedures address the standards required by its accrediting body. Home care agencies that are part of a larger organization will implement their parent organization's policies and procedures as applicable. The home care agency may need to develop additional policies and procedures specific to the agency while supporting the policies and procedures of the larger organization. Refer to Chapter 8 for a discussion on standards of practice.

Policies Related to Client Safety   In addition to, or as part of, its policies and procedures, the home care agency will develop processes to improve client safety. The Joint Commission (JC) has developed national client safety goals. Home care agencies that are accredited by the JC are required to review these goals and develop a response for each goal applicable to the scope of services provided. The response may be a policy, procedure, and/or process that outlines how the agency will meet each applicable safety goal. The JC's national client safety goals are reviewed and updated periodically (JCAHO, 2004).

All policies and procedures are reviewed at least annually by the advisory board and are revised as needed. The governing body is ultimately responsible for the approval of agency policies and procedures. The leadership team is responsible for assuring that the agency's policies and procedures are communicated to all staff and implemented throughout the home care agency.

Planning, Designing, and Providing Services

The home care agency leadership team defines in writing the scope of services that the agency will provide. These services may include skilled nursing, home health aide services, physical therapy, occupational therapy, speech therapy, medical social work, and supplies and equipment necessary to provide care. Additionally, some agencies may choose to provide nutrition consultation, pastoral care, volunteer services, in-home aide services, private duty (continuous care) services, home infusion pharmacy, and home medical equipment. The scope of services that a home care agency will provide is determined by assessing the (1) community's needs and expectations for services, (2) human resources available to provide the services, (3) licensure or regulatory limitations on the services the agency provides, (4) potential financial impact of providing the services, and (5) agency mission, vision, and goals.

Providing Services

Once an agency's scope of services is determined, the leadership team will decide how the home care agency will deliver each of the services defined in its scope of services. The leaders may choose to provide the service either through its own employees or contract with another entity to provide the service on its behalf under a contracted arrangement. At a minimum, the Medicare-certified home care agency must provide at least one of the core services previously defined wholly through its own employees.

Provision of Resources

The leadership team must provide the necessary resources to meet the home care agency's mission, vision, and goals, and provide the care defined in its scope of services. Areas that the leaders must continually assess include the agency's resource needs for space, equipment, and people. Space requirements for a home care agency usually include space for meetings, medical supplies, biohazardous waste, equipment cleaning, telecommunications equipment, computer equipment, administrative functions, and charting space for staff members who provide the home care services.

Equipment needs of a home care agency include telecommunications equipment (phones, beepers, cell phones); computers (servers, desktop computers, laptops); medical supplies; and medical equipment (scales, blood pressure cuffs, thermometers, bags, biohazardous waste containers, glucometers, and telehealth monitors). The leadership team must also assure that the agency has basic business resources available such as insurance, bonding, mechanisms for providing criminal background checks of employees, and any business licenses or certifications that may be required for it to do business.

Human resource needs of a home care agency include the leadership team, clerical support staff, billing staff, and staff to provide the care outlined in the agency's scope of services. At a minimum, a Medicare-certified home care agency must provide nursing and at least one other discipline such as physical therapy, speech therapy, home health aide services, occupational therapy, or medical social work.

Staffing Plans and the Provision of Care

The leadership team develops a staffing plan to assure that the home care agency has the appropriate staff available to provide its services. Areas the leadership team considers include the *right* number and *right* qualifications of staff available as well as the right scheduling of staff to meet the projected need for each service. An agency's client census and acuity levels change frequently, making it necessary for the leadership team to continually assess the home care agency's staffing plan.

The leaders provide the resources necessary for staff to provide for the care needs of the home care agency's clients. In addition to the provision of physical resources such as medical supplies, documentation materials, support staff, and equipment, the leaders assure that all staff members receive an orientation and training appropriate to their position. Initial orientation and training includes at a minimum a review of the home care agency's policies and procedures, Medicare Conditions of Participation for home health agencies, applicable licensure rules, service coverage and reimbursement guidelines, infection control and hand hygiene, employee and client safety, emergency management, and spiritual and cultural aspects of providing care. Teaching and learning methods should also be a component of home care staff orientation and ongoing education.

Home care staff provides client education on several levels as part of the home care admission. Staff education and competency in teaching are necessary for successful outcomes in home care. Effective staff will determine their clients' preferred learning methods along with any barriers that may impede the learning process. Common barriers to learning are lack of language and reading skills and hearing loss. Staff also provides education to clients regarding their rights and responsibilities as clients, home safety, emergency management, and disease management and prevention. The home care agency's leaders make available to staff current references and client education materials appropriate to the scope of care provided and the agency's client population. Resources are allocated for ongoing staff training on a continuing basis.

Information Management Planning

The home care agency leadership team develops an information management plan that provides a mechanism for coordination of client care. The plan provides assurance of a standardized format for the maintenance of information, and it details the agency's plan for backup and recovery of data in the event of a systems failure resulting in loss of data. The information plan defines the mechanisms for staff to coordinate care throughout the agency and with others involved in the client care such as staff conferences, e-mail, and documentation systems. The information plan also defines personnel access to certain levels or types of information in the home care agency. The need for access to information is based on the need for information to perform job functions.

Within the information plan is a contingency plan that addresses failure of the data system. The contingency plan allows agency functions to continue with the least amount of disruption in the case of a data system failure. The contingency plan also includes identifying provisions for backup and, if needed, reconstruction of lost electronic data.

Emergency Management Planning

The development of an emergency management plan for the home care agency is also a responsibility of the leadership team. The emergency management plan contains a proactive assessment of potential events that might occur that could result in interruption to agency operations and the provision of client care.

Disruption of home care services may result from many events and may affect both clients and staff. Examples of such events include adverse weather conditions such as hurricanes, flooding, and snow and ice storms; sickness such a flu epidemic; and major accidents such as an airplane crash with multiple casualties. Examples of major catastrophic events are terrorist attacks, nuclear disasters, war, and earthquakes.

In developing the emergency management plan, the home care agency's leaders must consider and plan how the agency will provide for the continuity of care for its clients. The leaders develop a system that prioritizes clients, communicates with staff and clients when usual channels of communication are interrupted, arranges for an alternate site for staff offices, and identifies community resources that may provide temporary care to the home care agency's clients.

Home care agencies that are part of a larger organization may coordinate their emergency management planning with their parent organization. The leaders assure that the emergency management plan is communicated to all staff, and that staff is provided with client educational materials that will instruct the agency's clients on what to do in the event of an emergency.

Practice drills that provide staff members with the opportunity to test their response in the event of an actual emergency are helpful and are usually planned by the leadership team. The Joint Commission recommends that the leadership team evaluate the agency response to the drills or to an actual emergency (JCAHO, 2004).

Strategic Planning

Strategic planning provides the home care leaders with a mechanism to plan for the future of the home care agency. Although many home care agencies will conduct an annual strategic planning session, strategic planning in the successful organization is an ongoing process. Often, as part of the strategic planning process, the leaders will perform a formal or informal review of the home care agency's perceived strengths and weaknesses, along with its potential opportunities and threats that may impact its successful performance. This is referred to as a SWOT (strengths, weaknesses, opportunities, and threats) analysis.

Examples of areas considered for examination during strategic planning include the following:

- Home care agency mission, vision, and goals.
- Overall effectiveness and performance of the current scope of services and any special programs currently provided by the agency.
- Needs of the current clients and staff to provide or improve the provision of the current scope of services, including consideration of the community and its referral sources and the position of the agency within the community relative to its competitors.
- Industry trends.
- Human resource needs, availability, and ability to recruit and retain qualified staff.
- Technology.

- Financial resources available to the agency.
- Regulatory and accreditation requirements.

The strategic plan is developed to support the agency's mission, vision, and goals based upon the leadership team's review and assessment of the relevant factors. The plan is then written and communicated throughout the agency.

Plans for implementation of the strategic plan are also the responsibility of the leadership team. The implementation plan should include objectives and goals, specific assignments to key personnel, expected deliverables, and a timeframe for completion. The leaders monitor the implementation plan and modify the plan as necessary to accomplish the agency's goals.

Results of the strategic plan are monitored. As part of the plan, the leaders determine how the success of the plan will be measured. The team then identifies data elements to collect, trend, and analyze. The data is then used to assess the success of the plan or to identify areas that may require revisions to the plan. When the data indicates a less than desired outcome or result, the leaders will reevaluate the area and take appropriate action. Action may include changes to current practice or, in some cases, elimination of the item from the agency's scope of services or operational plan. The measurement cycle of data collection, trending, analysis, and action will then be repeated to measure the impact of the plan revisions.

Annual Program Evaluation

An overall evaluation of the agency's total home care program is conducted annually. Participants in evaluation are the group of professional personnel appointed by the governing body or a subcommittee of this group, staff of the home care agency, consumers, and professional people outside of the agency working in conjunction with consumers. At a minimum, the program evaluation consists of an overall review of the agency operations including policies and procedures, client care, and agency administration. Individual state laws and regulations governing home care agencies may specify additional components to be included in the annual program evaluation. All areas are evaluated for effectiveness, efficiency, adequacy, and appropriateness.

Evaluation of Scope of Care

The evaluation addresses the entire scope of care and services provided by the home care agency, including services provided on its behalf by other entities. Data is collected and made available for analysis and assessment as part of the review. Data collected for assessment may include the following:

- Financial data, including costs of providing goods such as medical supplies and services, and the business mix (the proportion of the agency's revenue that is attributable to each service).
- Statistical data, including admissions, discharges, top diagnosis of agency clients, referrals (admitted and non-admitted), geographic distribution of customers, discharge disposition, and client outcomes.
- Performance improvement data, including client outcomes, client and staff satisfaction, performance improvement team priorities, risk management, infection control, and safety (staff and client incidents and accidents).

- Policy and procedure data, including the number and subjects of policies and procedures revised or developed throughout the year to support the agency's operation and activities of the policy and procedure committee if present in the agency.

Evaluation of Client Care

The evaluation of client care may be performed through review of the results of a quarterly medical record review. At least quarterly, a group of professional personnel representing the scope of services provided by the home care agency review a selection of clinical records. Records selected for review include both active and discharged or closed records representative of the services provided by the agency both directly by agency staff and through contracted arrangements during the quarter. The records are reviewed for "consistency with professional practice standards . . . and the agency's policies and procedures, compliance with the plan of care, the appropriateness, adequacy, and effectiveness of the services offered, and evaluations of anticipated client outcomes" (CMS, 2004d).

Financial Planning and Management

Annually, the leaders prepare an overall financial plan and budget. Generally accepted accounting principles guide the budget process. The plan includes an operating budget and a capital expenditure plan. The operating budget includes anticipated revenue and anticipated operating expenses. Operating expenses include the daily costs of doing business such as salaries, benefits, office supplies, rent, utilities, medical supplies, automobile expenses, and printing of forms and other materials. A capital expenditure plan to address both short-term and long-term capital needs is an additional component of the budget and financial plan for the agency. A long-term capital expenditure plan is developed to assess and plan for large (greater than $600,000 per single item) anticipated capital expenses that the agency expects to incur over at least the next three-year period. The long-term capital plan addresses how the agency will finance the costs of these items. Examples of items that could be included in a long-term capital expenditure plan are new construction projects or the purchase of a new information system. Short-term or lower-cost capital items may be included in the annual budget. Examples of these capital items include copiers, fax machines, and computers (CMS, 2004b).

Prospective Payment System

Home care agencies that are certified to provide services to Medicare beneficiaries are paid by a prospective payment system (PPS). The system, resulting from the implementation of the Balanced Budget Act of 1997, was enacted in October 2000. Under the system, Medicare pays home health agencies a predetermined base payment. The payment is adjusted according to the differences in wages across the country and the client's condition, care needs, and service needs. Collectively, this is referred to as the case-mix adjustment. The prospective payment system enters into the financial plan of home care agencies (CMS, 2005).

Development of the Financial Plan

The process followed to develop the financial plan and budget may vary between agencies. Some governing bodies direct a top-down approach where the budget is provided to the leaders. Other governing bodies use a bottom-up approach soliciting input from lower-level staff up through the leaders to the governing body. Most financial plans and budgets are developed using a combination of input from the leaders, past financial performance, market factors, and anticipated growth.

Budget Formats

Budget formats may also differ. A small agency may have a simple financial plan and budget while a detailed, complex financial plan and budget may be necessary for a large agency. The budget of an agency that is part of a larger organization such as a hospital may find its budget incorporated into the larger organization's budget. In this case, the home care agency's budget and capital expenditure plan must be clearly displayed within the larger budget and financial plan documents.

Once completed and approved by the governing body, the leaders will use the financial plan and budget to help guide the operations of the agency. Actual performance, revenue, and expenses must be continually monitored and compared to the budget. Variances between the budget and the actual financial performance may develop. If a negative variance occurs, adjustments must be made to either the expenses or the budget to ensure the ongoing viability of the agency. A positive variance may help to support unanticipated growth. If the agency has projects in its long-term capital expenditure plan, the leaders monitor performance and progress towards these goals.

The budget and financial plan should ultimately support the agency's provision of its scope of services to accomplish its mission, vision, and goals. Regardless of the methods used to develop the budget and financial plan, or the format used to document the budget and plan, successful financial plans and budgets are easily understood, usable, and communicated to those responsible for their implementation, and then continually monitored and modified as needed.

Contracts

A home care agency may use contracts to assist it in the provision of services or to realize revenue for the budget. There are several types of contractual arrangements. Preferred provider contracts are common where a payer for services, usually an insurance company, enters into an agreement with the home care agency. Preferred provider services that are provided to its enrollees are often offered at reduced rates. The agency may enter into contracts for goods such as equipment or medical supplies or services to provide on behalf of others or to be provided. These last two contractual arrangements will be discussed in more detail in this section.

Contracts with Other Entities

The leaders may choose to provide services through contracts with other entities that will provide services on its behalf. The reasons for contracting for services vary. The home care agency may not have the volume of business in a particular service to make hiring and maintaining staff in that area economically feasible. Conversely, the agency may have too much volume in a service area for its own staff to manage and contracts with a provider to supplement its own staff. Regardless of the reason for contracting with another provider, the contract between the two entities must contain certain elements required by certification and accreditation bodies.

These elements include the scope and location of services to be provided, financial arrangements, provision that the ultimate ownership and responsibility for the client and service lies with the home care agency, terms of the agreement, record-keeping, confidentiality, and responsibilities for scheduling, care planning, and coordination of care. Before signing, all contracts should be reviewed by the agency's legal counsel. Once a contract is signed and implemented, the home care agency leaders provide oversight and monitoring of the contracted services. This oversight and monitoring may be performed on multiple levels as part of the clinical record review process, the annual agency program evaluation, and during the contract renewal process.

Contract to Provide Services

The home care agency may also enter into a contract arrangement with another entity whereby the home care agency will provide services for the other entity. In this scenario, the agency leadership has the responsibility to meet the terms of the contract. If the home care agency is accredited by an accrediting body such as the JC, that body may also assess whether the agency has provided services to meet the terms of the contract as part of the accrediting process. Again, the home care agency's legal counsel should review all contracts before they are signed.

Many legal, licensure, certification, and accreditation standards factors are taken into consideration when deciding to enter or not to enter into a contractual arrangement. Potential contracts must include all required elements. Review by legal counsel is strongly recommended prior to signing any contract for the agency.

Quality Management and Performance Improvement

The leaders plan and direct the quality management and performance improvement activities of the agency. Quality improvement priorities are identified to improve client care outcomes; reduce risks to the agency; improve client, staff, and referral source satisfaction with the agency; and increasingly, assure compliance with applicable laws and regulations.

Performance Improvement Plan

A performance improvement plan is necessary for home care organizations to monitor and upgrade services and to remain competitive in their choice of services. The plan, developed by the leadership team, describes the performance improvement program components, the methodology that the agency will follow to accomplish its performance improvement goals, the potential data sources for identification of priorities, and plans for displaying and communicating data and results of performance improvement activities. The leaders are responsible for allocating adequate resources to meet the goals outlined in the plan. There are many potential data sources that leaders may use to identify performance improvement priorities. Some of the data sources are satisfaction survey results (client, staff, physician, and referral sources); incident and accident statistics; infection-control data; results of clinical record reviews; publicly reported outcomes such as the JC Quality Check, CMS Adverse Outcome

Reports, CMS Outcome Based Quality Improvement (OBQ) Reports, and CMS Home Care Compare; claims denial rates; and utilization data. Refer to Chapter 10 for a detailed discussion on performance improvement.

Compliance Plan

Initiatives to combat fraud and abuse in the Medicare and Medicaid programs have been implemented by the federal government. The Office of Inspector General (OIG) has published a model home health agency compliance plan that home care agencies may use as a reference guide. The OIG model plan includes recommendations for policies, procedures, staff training, and monitoring, and plan evaluation activities to prevent fraud and abuse in an agency. Using the OIG model, a compliance plan should be established by the leadership team for their home care agency. In addition to the model plan, the OIG publishes an annual departmental work plan that outlines areas the OIG staff will focus on for their fraud and abuse initiatives in the coming year. This work plan should be used by leaders to identify the home care agency's compliance monitoring and training activities (HHS Office of Inspector General, 2004).

Summary

The basic functions of home care agency leadership have been outlined in this chapter. Although these functions will remain constant, how the leadership team manages the components of each function will vary. The leadership must continually assess changes in customer needs, market factors, technology, coverage and reimbursement guidelines, accreditation standards, and availability of qualified staff. In response, leaders continually monitor, assess, reevaluate, and make changes to agency services and programs to meet these challenges.

References

Centers for Medicare and Medicaid Services Conditions of Participation for Home Health Agencies. (2004a). *Medicare interpretive guidelines for home health agencies.* Standard 484.14(b).

Centers for Medicare and Medicaid Services Conditions of Participation for Home Health Agencies. (2004b). *Medicare interpretive guidelines for home health agencies.* Standard 484.4.

Centers for Medicare and Medicaid Services Conditions of Participation for Home Health Agencies. (2004c). *Medicare interpretive guidelines for home health agencies of registered nurses.* Standard 484.14d.

Centers for Medicare and Medicaid Services Conditions of Participation for Home Health Agencies. (2004d). *Medicare interpretive guidelines for home health agencies.* Standard 484.14(i).

Centers for Medicare and Medicaid Services. (2005). *Home Health PPS.* Retrieved January, 13, 2006, from
http://www.cms.hhs.gov/homeHealthPPS/01-overview.asp

Health & Human Services Office of Inspector General. (2004). *Compliance program guidance for home health agencies.* Retrieved September 17, 2004, from

http://www.oig.hhs.gov/fraud/complianceguidance.html/04

Joint Commission on the Accreditation of Healthcare Organizations. (1999). *Using performance measurement to improve outcomes in home care and hospice settings.* Oakbrook Terrace: Author.

Joint Commission on the Accreditation of Healthcare Organizations. (2004). *JCAHO home care standards manual.* Retrieved September 9, 2004, from

http://www.jcaho.org/accredited+organizations/behavioral+health+care/npsg/04

Sherman, R. O. (2005). Growing our future nursing leaders. *Nursing Administration Quarterly,* *29*(2), 125-132.

Chapter 8

Legal Issues

Jeanie Stoker, RN, MPA, BC

Key Terms

Advance Directives	Nurse Practice Acts	Scope of Practice
Malpractice	Nursing Practice	Standards of Practice
Negligence		

L egal concerns, regulatory mandates, and legislative issues are concerns of all businesses; health care is no exception. In addition to federal and state legislation, the health care industry must also adhere to issues related to licensure. Because health care is a service industry that is related to life-and-death situations, there are some issues that become emotion-ridden, especially to health care providers and clients.

One of the current legal issues that face health care providers and organizations is the malpractice crisis (Newfield, 2005). Even the best practitioner can be sued for any care provided or not provided, but by using a proactive approach and by being aware of state and federal regulations, some of these situations can be prevented. This chapter addresses the legal issues that should be familiar to nurses practicing in home care.

Nursing Practice and Licensure

Nursing practice, broadly defined, is the performance of skills and services for the purpose of assisting people in the pursuit of wellness, or through illness and/or death. Levels of nursing practice include advanced practice nurses, registered nurses, and practical nurses. Each state's Board of Nursing regulates the practice of nursing, which requires licensure.

A Brief History of Licensure

Professional licensure is the legal process that grants permission for a qualified person to practice in a certain jurisdiction in which it would be illegal to do so without a license. Licenses are issued by government agencies. For nurses, the governing agency is each state's Board of Nursing. The qualified person who is eligible to become licensed as a nurse must have graduated from a nursing program, or is a nurse who holds a license in another state. Upon successful completion of a nursing program, the nursing student becomes a graduate nurse. Graduate nurses then become eligible to take the state board examination. Upon passing the state board examination, the graduate nurse becomes licensed. Nursing schools prepare students to be licensed as practical nurses or registered nurses. Thus the nurse is a licensed practical nurse (LPN) or a licensed registered nurse (RN). State boards of nursing regulate both levels of nursing.

Physicians and dentists were the first professionals to be licensed, with nurses generally the next licensed professionals. In 1903, North Carolina became the first state to develop a "nurse registration act" (Brent, 2001, p. 302). This laid the blueprint for other states, so that by 1923 all states had developed **nurse practice acts.** Nurse practice acts "define the practice of nursing, give guidance within the scope of practice issues, and set standards for the nursing profession" (Guido, 2006, p. 224). **Scope of practice** legally refers to "permissible boundaries of practice for the health professional as defined by rules and regulations" (Guido, 2006, p. 238).

In the early years of nursing, registration was not mandatory, but those who did register with the state were allowed to use "RN" behind their name. During this time the predetermined requirements and practice guidelines were minimal or completely non-existent. Physicians sat on the nursing boards and enforced what rules were in place while promoting their perceived direction for nursing.

New York State changed the direction of nursing in 1938 by establishing the first mandatory nurse practice act. New York was very progressive in establishing two levels of nursing, the registered nurse (RN) and the licensed practical nurse (LPN), sometimes called licensed vocational nurse (LVN), and defined nursing practices at both levels. New York also propagated the nursing profession's autonomy by establishing nursing boards that were composed of nurses and not physicians.

In 1911, the American Nurses Association was founded and a new definition of nursing was established (Christy, 1969, p. 38). Unfortunately, the definition was very restrictive in the nurse's role of diagnostic and therapeutic interventions. This statement was not truly expanded until 1971, when nursing specialties needed to expand their scope of practice to meet the intent of their new roles. Again, New York led the way by changing its regulations to include such definitions as nursing diagnosis and joint practice (Brent, 2001).

Today the practice of nursing has evolved and allows greater autonomy, especially as more nursing care is delivered away from acute care setting into home care, community health, and long-term care (Guido, 2006). Each state has developed very specific guidelines and definitions related to the scope of nursing practice. Because of the wide degree of variance in each state, it is critical that all nurses review and understand their state's practice act. Because change in these practice acts usually requires legislative intervention, it is also imperative that nurses stay abreast of new proposals and changes that are introduced on the federal and state levels, as this is an ever-changing area.

Nurse Practice Acts

Nurse practice acts are the rules and laws that define the practice of nursing in each state. The rules range from scope of practice to supervisory oversight to educational guidelines. It is imperative that all nurses obtain a copy of the practice act for each state in which they hold a license.

The practice acts in each state, while different, cover similar subjects. These usually include, but are not limited to, the following:

- Definitions.
- Empowerment of the Board of Nursing for regulatory oversight of the practice as well as the rules.
- Development of the board, including members, bylaws, and standard operating procedures.
- Establishment of fees.
- Licensure guidelines including endorsement, examination, and reciprocity.
- Licensure renewal process.
- Delineation of nurses, such as the licensed practical nurse, registered nurse, and the advanced nurse practitioner.
- Disciplinary guidelines, processes, and outcomes.
- Rules regulating the suspension, revocation, and retirement of licenses.
- Nursing institution requirements, guidelines, and processes.
- Continuing education requirements and rules.
- Other laws and regulations as mandated by the state.

This general overview of the details included in nursing practice acts does vary from state to state. Each state has a written document that will provide the licensed nurse with the rules and regulations required by law to be a practicing clinician in that state.

Standards of Practice

All nursing practice settings have **standards of practice** that are the "levels or degrees of quality considered adequate by a given profession. Standards of practice are the skills and learning commonly possessed by members of a profession" (Guido, 2006, p. 55). Standards of clinical nursing practice include both standards of care and standards of professional performance. Standards of practice are determined by many different means, including the nurse practice acts of each state, professional organizations like the American Nurses Association (ANA) and the National League for Nursing (NLN), specialty organizations like the Association of Operating Room Nurses (AORN), federal organizations like the Joint Commission (JC), the policies of the institution in which the nurse is employed, and the role or job description of the nurse (ANA, 1999; Guido, 2006).

The delivery of quality nursing care demands that each nursing discipline meet its individual standards of practice. Home care nurses need to know the standards in their practice setting. There are specifically defined responsibilities and expectations for nurses such as the supervision of a home care aide as defined by the Medicare Conditions of Participation. Home care nurses are liable for their actions as well as the actions of those under their supervision. The RN develops a care plan in accordance with the physician's orders. She then directs the LPN, LVN, home care aide, and other practitioners in the care of the client. In the event that an injury or death occurs, the RN may be held liable for all her actions as well as actions of those she supervises.

Regulatory Agents

In each state, the nurse practice act is the "Bible" of nursing practice and the State Board of Nursing is the regulatory body that enforces the law. The state government usually appoints key board members and approves nursing law, but other regulatory bodies govern nursing.

The federal laws that regulate nursing as well as all health care delivery are the Medicare laws. The laws include *Conditions of Participation for Home Care Agencies, and Hospice Manual for Medicare-Certified Hospices.* All Medicare providers have regulations developed by the Centers for Medicare and Medicaid Services (CMS), which establish the conditions of participation.

The conditions of participation provide rules for home care that impact nursing in the following areas:

- Client rights and responsibilities
- Personnel qualifications and clinical competencies
- Documentation
- Complaint and grievance processes
- Confidentiality
- Clinical assessment
- Compliance with professional standards and principles
- Skilled nursing services and duties
- Supervision guidelines
- Coordination of client care
- Physician order obtainment and review
- Home care aide training and skill assessment
- Policy development and review
  (CMS, 2005.)

The state's key regulatory role was defined in the licensure area. Other state practices may also overlap in the nursing area. In home care, the board for social workers as well as the board of pharmacy and possibly the board of medicine influence nursing practice and the rules required to practice.

The Joint Commission (JC) is not a regulatory body but rather an accrediting body whose mission is "to continuously improve the safety and quality of care provided to the public through the provision of health care accreditation and related services that support performance improvement in health care organizations" (JCAHO, 2004, p. 1). Because of its focus, nursing plays a pivotal role in the accrediting process, and thus has many processes that are dictated by the standards developed by the JC. Nurses need to review these standards as well as participate in the ongoing accreditation process. Although Medicare and state licensure surveys are usually conducted every 18 to 36 months, today health care institutions are working with staff to insure ongoing compliance and readiness with the survey standards.

In today's health care environment, the RN is inundated with rules, regulations, documentation, and client care. In home care typically an RN will carry a caseload of clients. Several staff members may be involved with the clients' care in that nurse's caseload. For this reason, because it cannot be assumed that all team members are providing care as ordered and directed, it is the responsibility of the RN to insure that compliance is occurring. This is accomplished through review of the original doctor's orders with all caregivers, direct observation and supervision, and reporting. All RNs must know the required state and federal standards, including competencies, and the policies and procedures of their employment agencies.

The nurse also has a responsibility to provide care at a standard recognized by any other home care nurse. Sometimes this expectation is ambiguous; an example is wound care protocols. In many areas today, what constitutes proper wound care is a question not easily answered. There has been a recent increase of litigation in some areas where home care clients who have chronic pain due to long-term wounds are receiving large settlements based on improper practice (Newfield, 2005). Dailey and Newfield (2005) offer suggestions to home care agencies that may reduce regulatory and legal exposure such as developing procedures and policies that reflect current research (best practice), education for personnel on proper documentation and wound categorization, and client advocacy.

Nurses who are concerned about any orders they are asked to implement must be sure to know whom they can go to for support and direction. The Wound, Ostomy, Continence Nurses Society (WOCN) has some of the most up-to-date research and proactive guidelines in the industry. This information should be reviewed and shared with both agency supervisors and medical directors. Nurses need to be proactive in the pursuit of appropriate practice. Not only is this the best for the client, but it will strengthen the nurse's defense if that ever becomes necessary.

Client Rights

The importance and necessity of respect, knowledge, and action related to the rights of clients in the health care system is succinctly stated by Pozgar (2001): "The continuing trend of consumer awareness, coupled with increased governmental regulations, makes it advisable for caregivers to understand the scope of [client] rights and how to ensure them" (p. 322).

Patient's Bill of Rights

In 1997, then-President Clinton signed into law the Patient's Bill of Rights. The Bill of Rights identifies clients' rights as well as their responsibilities. There are three key goals: strengthening consumer confidence in the health care system, promoting strong relationships between the client and the health care professional, and promoting consumer responsibility for safeguarding his or her own health. These rights include:

- The right to information. Understandable information allows consumers to make informed decisions.
- The right to choose. Clients must have access to the provider and specialist. This includes women's right to OB-GYN services.
- Access to emergency services. All clients have the right to emergency care when acute situations occur.
- Being a full partner in health care decisions. Clients have the right to participate in their health care decisions and have an appropriate representative to decide on their behalf when they are unable to.

- Care without discrimination. Clients must be treated respectfully and equally regardless of age, race, ethnicity, religion, or source of payment.
- The right to privacy. Each person has the right to confidentiality.
- The right to speedy complaint resolution. Health care consumers should be able to voice a complaint when they feel services are substandard and to expect follow-up resolution that is fair and timely.
- Responsibility. With rights come client responsibility. Clients are expected to be active participants in health promotion as well as decision making.

In the home care setting, clients are also provided a document that details their individual rights and responsibilities. Additional rights include ethical standards and conduct, absence of abuse, clear communication, and a hotline number to report concerns or complaints. Home care nurses need to review this document with their clients and families upon the client's admission to home care and throughout the service period. The RN must also insure that all caregivers—professional, paraprofessional, lay, and family—respect and honor these rights.

Health Insurance Portability and Accountability Act (HIPAA)

In 1997, the Health Insurance Portability and Accountability Act (HIPAA) provided additional rights for clients that insure confidentiality. The provisions include the following:

- Privacy. Health care organizations must inform clients that they do have privacy rights, including how their medical information is being used by the organization.
- Transactions. These are a set of standards that allow for information to be shared between entities. This allows payers and providers to communicate in a uniform way.
- Code sets. Consistent code sets provide a universal language that will reduce redundancy and cost.
- Security. Although confidentiality has always been expected in the health care setting, HIPAA mandates specific processes and penalties. Besides protection of confidential information, these processes require additional safeguards for anticipated threats and hazards that may compromise the integrity of the information, unauthorized use or disclosure of information, and a compliance plan that insures that all rules are followed.
- Unique identifiers. The last provision requires that all clients, providers, and employers have a unique national identifier.

Although these are the key focus areas of HIPAA, today the most important focus for the home care nurse is the "privacy notice." It is mandatory that this document be given to all clients in a covered entity, which includes home care. The core focus of the privacy notice is to provide clients with information about the following:

- Their rights under HIPPA.
- Access to their medical records.
- Their medical treatment, including how information is used.
- Finances related to their medical situation.
- Information on how to make a complaint. This section should include a local phone number as well as a phone number and the address of the Office of Civil Rights.

Confidentiality

The most appropriate way for health care workers to handle information that becomes known to them through their work is to treat all information as confidential. Home care providers, by virtue of entering the private residents of their clients, are exposed to more private and personal information than is usual in the acute care setting. Confidentiality goes beyond client information; it includes information about a client's family, home life, and the condition of the home. Confidentiality also includes records, both paper and electronic.

A breach of confidentiality does not occur when client information is shared among members of the health care team who are also involved in the client's care. The client must sign a release of information form before information is released to third-party payors (Guido, 2006).

Client   Nurses involved in client care have been educated in issues related to clients' rights to privacy and as such have respected their privacy. In home care, this respect extends to include respect for clients' homes. Many homes are not as clean or maintained as well as health care personnel would like; nevertheless, the home is to be respected. Recently an experienced nurse brought an orienting nurse with her on an admission visit. Upon arrival, the experienced nurse asked the client for permission to sit in a dirty, torn chair as well as moving a pile of old newspapers so she could put her home care bag down. When they completed the visit, the inexperienced nurse commented on the request, as it was such a dreadful area. The nurse stated, "yes, the place was not a place I would bring my family, but it was all the client had and very important to her. The torn chair was her luxury, and I will honor it as I would a queen's throne."

Records   The medical record contains the client's personal data, insurance data, medical history, reports of all tests, and anecdotal notes of all health care providers who have been involved with the client's care. Health facilities own the health records of the clients they serve. Generally, a client has the right to all of the information in their record, and may ask to have a copy of the record. A facility may charge a fee for this service.

The medical record is confidential and may not be shared with others including family members without the consent of the client. Health care providers are bound to respect the confidentiality of medical records including records that are stored in computers. Usually health care personnel must use a password before accessing a client record that is electronically stored.

Informed Consent

Clients have the right to make decisions based on explanations regarding their disease process, treatment, choices, and outcomes. Failure to obtain informed consent prior to health care intervention could be grounds for assault, battery, or neglect. A focus of informed consent is ensuring that the client is competent enough to provide an informed consent. A person may be declared incompetent via a physician's declaration, a legal proceeding, or in a specific situation. The nurse who obtains the informed consent should document that the client is alert and oriented and is aware of current events and situations. Each state has its own definition and process for declaring incompetence and the actions that should be completed if the client is determined to be incompetent. For example, in South Carolina, two physicians are required to sign that a person is incompetent before the next of kin may sign the consent on the client's behalf. The two types of informed consent are written and implied.

Written Consent   Home care clients sign an initial consent for all home care services and disciplines. In urgent situations, clients may only be able to verbalize their consent, but in the home care setting the written consent is the norm.

Implied Consent   Implied consent, when the client is only able to verbalize consent, also includes the acceptance of routine care that usually does not require a legal document. A nursing example of implied consent is when a nurse explains to a client that she is about to take his vital signs and he allows it.

Informed Refusal

Health care consumers have the right to refuse care or service. Informed refusal may either be written or implied. When an individual does not want a specific procedure performed and he verbally expresses such, the health care practitioner cannot force it on him. There are certain elements that make refusal an informed refusal. These elements, which must be clarified and documented, are the following:

- The refusal must be voluntary, so that the client does not feel coerced or threatened.
- The client must be made aware of the consequences of the refusal.
- The client must be competent to make the decision.

The home care nurse must document these points and when appropriate, communicate them to the attending physician. Clients should be told that refusal of care or treatment may lead to early discharge. As with all issues, physician awareness and early discharge must be documented.

Patient Self-Determination Act

The Patient Self-Determination Act was signed into law in 1990. There were three basic purposes for this act:

1. Clients who are informed of their rights are more likely to take advantage of them.
2. If clients are more actively involved in decisions about their medical care, then that care will be more responsive to their needs.
3. Clients may choose care that is less costly.
   (Rouse, 1991, p. 21.)

In 1996, Medicare required home care agencies as well as hospitals, nursing homes, HMOs, and hospices receiving Medicare funds to implement the following:

1. Establish written policies and procedures concerning the right of adult clients to informed consent and refusal of treatment. All clients must be informed of these policies.
2. Inform clients of their rights under state law, including the use of advance directives to make decisions regarding treatment and nontreatment.
3. Determine the existence of advance directives and document them into the medical record.
4. Insure that care or services provided are not compromised or the client is not discriminated against due to the existence of, or lack of, advance directives.
5. Comply and honor advance directives in accordance with state practice laws.
6. Provide educational programs regarding the law and advance directives.
   (Duffy, 2001.)

Advance Directives   People who have made decisions about their medical care, prior to their actually needing the care, are said to have made their wishes known in advance of need. Theses wishes are collectively known as **advance directives.** Since the passage of the

Patient Self-Determination Act, most health care professionals have had contact with advance directives either through their own self-reflection about end-of-life issues, or through discussions and guidance with clients and families with health care decisions or support of their end-of-life decisions. Usually advance directives are used to refuse certain treatments; however, the directives may be used to request treatments. Advance Directives are legally binding and come in several formats (Ramsey & Mitty, 2003).

Living Will   The living will provides a written mechanism to establish an individual's wishes for end-of-life treatment or the forgoing of specific treatment. In order for a living will to be implemented, the client must have completed the will as a competent adult but be currently in a permanent vegetative state, in an unconscious state, or diagnosed with a terminal illness. The usual treatment options include the provision or withholding of blood products, hydration, artificial nutrition, and surgery or other invasive procedures including cardiopulmonary resuscitation (CPR). Individuals may also add specific requests and directions.

Home care nurses must ask their clients, upon admission, if they have a living will. If a client has a living will, the nurse should obtain a copy and document its existence in the client's record. Key points of the living will should also be documented. If a living will does not exist, the agency must provide the client with education about living wills and the opportunity to complete one if desired. As with all advance directives, the client always has the right to change or revoke a living will.

Durable Power of Attorney for Health Care   A durable power of attorney for health care is a document that has been executed, witnessed, and signed. It provides for a designated individual (designee) to make health care decisions for the client if they become unable to make such decisions for themselves. As with all legal documents, the individual completing this directive must be a competent adult. The designee usually is a close family member, but this is not required. Nurses are often exempt from being the designee if they will be providing health care to the client.

Generally, a health care power of attorney is much broader than a living will, as it is not limited to terminal states or end-of-life care. The designee may also make decisions related to routine health care and services or their refusal. This document may also be changed or revocated as the client desires, and it generally provides the designee with immunity from civil, criminal, or disciplinary actions.

Home care nurses must ask their clients if they have a durable power of attorney, and if they do, the document, if activated, should be examined. A copy of the document is placed in the client's medical record. The home care nurse documents in the record the presence of the durable power of attorney and the identity of the designee.

Issues of Concern

There are several client issues of concern that demand constant vigilance and surveillance by home care providers. Although complex and sometimes difficult to identify, the most common issues are now discussed.

Negligence and Neglect

Negligence is "the failure to exercise the degree of care that a person of ordinary prudence would exercise under the same circumstances" (Duffy, 2001, p. 13). Negligence includes not doing something that should be done as well as doing something that should not have been done. Anyone could be deemed negligent. In health care when a nonprofessional is negligent, it is negligence; when a professional is negligent it is usually malpractice (Guido, 2006).

Neglect is defined as "the failure or omission of proper attention to a person or thing, whether inadvertent, negligent, or willful" (Brent, 2001, pp. 283–284). Abuse is actual mental or physical mistreatment. Although client neglect and abuse can occur in any setting, the client's home is the place where such actions usually occur, and are most often overlooked by health care personnel. Nurses should be aware that, although uncomfortable to admit, abuse and neglect often occurs at the hands of caregivers (Guido, 2006).

Neglect may be seen in the home when there are multiple caregivers or a caregiver who provides care to many people, including children. There may be reason for suspicion when the client has a loss of appetite or clinging behaviors. Constant soiled linens and undergarments as well as poor housekeeping should be assessed for potential neglect.

Malpractice

Malpractice as a term denotes a higher level of specificity than negligence. It refers to professional standards of care, and accordingly, the defendant must be a professional. "Courts have continually defined malpractice as any professional misconduct, unreasonable lack of skill, or fidelity in professional or judicial duties" (Guido, 2006, p. 72).

Home care staff often question suspicious bruising, abrasions, or fractures, but they are often remiss in identifying more subtle signs of abuse or neglect that are often confused with the aging process. Weight loss, withdrawal, constant complaints of pain, reports of frequent falls, or verbal outburst by the client or family are some abuse signs that are frequently missed.

Abuse

The National Center on Elder Abuse (1997), located in Washington, DC, researches and maintains statistics and trends related to elder abuse. The following statement has been retrieved from the center's website:

> Elder abuse in domestic settings is a serious problem, affecting hundreds of thousands of elderly people across the country. However, because it is still largely hidden in the shroud of family secrecy, elder abuse is grossly underreported. Some experts estimate that only 1 out of 14 domestic elder abuse incidents is reported. (National Center on Elder Abuse, 1997, p. 1.)

Abuse is not always physical in nature; abuse may also be verbal or financial. Some people will attempt to care for an elderly person and use their money to maintain the entire family. If this leads to poor care, or inadequate medications or food, then it is abuse. Abuse may also take the form of denying clients access to their money.

The home care provider has a legal and ethical obligation to report suspected abuse or neglect. Each state has specific departments and hotlines that can be contacted to report situations that may be abusive. Additionally, some state nurse practice acts require reporting of neglect and abuse. All health care providers should know the hotline phone number and the process for reporting abuse. Health care providers often overlook subtle abuse signs or feel the situation is the best possible or are afraid of retaliation against the client or employee. Anyone, including the client, can and should call when abuse or neglect is suspected. Clients should have the phone number of their home care agency and should be reminded by their home care nurse that they may call anytime. Often, reports can be done anonymously. Box 8-1 gives a partial list of signs and symptoms of client abuse.

BOX 8-1 SIGNS AND SYMPTOMS OF CLIENT ABUSE AND NEGLECT

- Skin breaks, bruises, welts, decubiti
- Poor body hygiene
- Soiled bedclothes
- Dry skin, tenting (dehydration)
- Hunger
- Weight loss
- Dirty environment
- No social contact for long periods of time
- Disappearance of personal items or clothes
- No input into use of personal finances

Home care providers should be educated about signs and symptoms of abuse as well as their responsibilities related to the abuse issue. Supervisors should respond to employee concerns by providing a second opinion, obtaining additional resources, and providing support. Reporting situations of abuse often lead to family disruption as well as discomfort for the staff. Ongoing litigation and court proceedings can monopolize staff and cause anxiety. Leadership will have to provide ongoing education and support for appropriate abuse reporting to be done as needed.

Abandonment

A home care agency may be charged with abandonment when a client's discharge is considered a unilateral decision or when the discharge is based on the client's inability to pay. As all nurses now know, discharge planning, whether in an acute care or long-term setting, begins during the admission process. The admitting home care nurse defines the client's plan of care using input from the client and the client's family. Once the plan of care is designed, then care continues until goals are met or services cannot be provided in accordance with agency policy and the safety of those involved. The home care RN needs to know the admission and discharge policy of the agency to insure that he or the agency is never charged with abandonment. One action that will support the discharge process is a physician's order, though it may not be required in all states and agencies.

A typical discharge policy may include discharging a client when:

1. All goals have been met.
2. The physician orders the discharge.
3. The family or client discharges the agency.
4. The client's homebound status is inconsistent with Medicare or other payor source requirements.
5. There is a safety risk to home care staff.
6. Another agency replaces the existing agency.
7. The client requires care greater than can be provided by the agency, such as 24-hour care.

Each agency will define in writing its discharge criteria. It is the responsibility of the home care RN to know the discharge guidelines.

Tele-Health

Forty years ago hospitals discovered that nurses were able to oversee more clients if the clients had individual monitors that monitored their vital signs and other key functions. By introducing cardiac, IV, and other monitors, nurses were able to care for those clients with the most urgent needs. Telemetry and step-down units have become routine in all acute care settings, and these services have eventually come to home care.

With the implementation of reimbursement based on diagnosis and services, agencies had to find better ways to maximize clinical efficiencies without compromising outcomes. Prior to the Medicare Prospective Payment System, home care agencies were reimbursed on a per-visit basis. This promoted inefficiencies, as agencies had incentives to see the client as much as possible. This was not necessarily a bad thing, as these visits did provide clinical assessment and teaching. Clients were educated quicker, and disease exacerbations were discovered sooner. However, with the reimbursement changes and the limited number of home care RNs, other mechanisms were needed. Enter the tele-health era of home care.

Tele-health services are provided in a variety of ways.

- Telephone. Some agencies have been successful in reducing on-site visits by having home care nurse and/or home care case managers call their clients and evaluate their needs and symptoms over the phone. Although the data obtained is subjective, many chronic conditions centers have noted reduced exacerbations and hospitalizations through these telephone interventions.

- Televideos. These systems provide on-site video cameras that allow observation from both parties. For example, nurses can view a wound and observe the wound care provided or review the insulin injection process to insure that the dose and administration are correct. The client can see his or her own nurse on the screen while receiving education and feedback (Russo, 2001).

- Internet. Clients may be able to access their agency via the Internet, cable, or other Web-based programs. These are newer systems, but the manufacturers tout early positive results. As clients are able to provide clinical information via this medium, the home care agency can intervene as needed (Tsai & Starren, 2001).

- Telemonitoring. Much like its inclient predecessor, these monitors provide daily data that allows the home care nurse to assess the client electronically. The monitors allow home care nurses to visit the client when they are needed, not just because the visit was scheduled. Early outcomes have shown a significant reduction in visits and reduced hospitalizations, especially in the congestive heart failure population (Tsai & Starren, 2001).

These are just a few examples of new technology that will support home care nurses. Although these systems are not intended to replace nurses' critical thinking skills, as daily data allow nurses to see the clients with greater needs, the systems help RNs maximize their abilities.

Nurses need to remember that they are still responsible for their clients and therefore should never rely solely on any electronic intervention. Although the technology does promote and allow fewer on-site interventions, RNs need to review all transmitted data on a regular basis to assess early warning signs and intervene appropriately.

Impact of the Legislative Process

The legislative process is the process by which legislation (laws) are enacted by both state and federal governmental bodies (senates and houses of congress or states). The process includes the introduction of a bill, the committee and floor action to be taken, the compromises, and once complete, the signing or rejection by the governor or the President of the United States. Once signed, the legislation becomes law, and is forwarded to an administrative agency such as the state Board of Nursing. The administrative agencies compile the rules that must be enacted at the each individual health care agency. In light of the multiple steps in the legislative process, the importance of early political action by nursing is vital to ensure that fair and appropriate laws, rules, and regulations are promulgated.

Nurses have been accused of political apathy (Des Jardin, 2001a, 2001b), but this author tends to believe that it is because nurses do not realize that they can take action and make a difference. Suggestions for action include:

- Write or e-mail your legislator. Identify the purpose of the letter and your view or concern about the issue. Provide factual evidence and statistics when possible. If possible, tell a true client story. Be sure to exclude all client information and just share the story. Legislators do want to know what is going on at home and how they can improve the quality of life of their constituents. Written letters, because they are personal, are always better than e-mail but use e-mail if it is the only resource available. Nurses have strong credibility and your story needs to be told.

- Call your representative. Local representatives have their numbers in the phone book and many also have their local and capitol numbers listed. In Washington, calling (202) 224-3121 will allow a person to ask for their state representative. When you call, you will talk with a legislative aide. It is fine to share your concern or story with them. They will pass on your information.

- Visit your congressperson either in Washington or your state capitol. Visit them in person. For best results, call ahead and make an appointment. Develop a small agenda and bring any supporting documentation with you. Share local newspaper or magazine stories. The more local and personal, the better. If you speak with the legislative aide, let them know your concerns and how much you appreciate their time. This is the best way to get your story heard.

- Become active in your professional and other organizations. Although nurses' expertise is in health care, nurses have a great opportunity to advocate for education, elder care, gun control, and many other issues. Masses influence the legislative process, and the more voices heard, the stronger the response. Get involved because you are the professional.

- Support a candidate. Get active in the election process. Find out which candidate shares your ideas and values, then host a fundraiser, volunteer to campaign, or offer a financial contribution.

- Seek public office. Nurses are needed on task forces, on government committees, and in the legislative arena. Many of these positions are appointed rather elected positions. Your professional nursing organization or party affiliation chapter can assist you with an election or an appointment.

- VOTE. All the other suggestions may seem overwhelming, but voting just takes a few minutes. Become informed and learn about all the candidates and issue. Voting is not a privilege but it is a civic responsibility, a true from of client advocacy. (Stoker, 2003).

It is amazing to see how many bills are related to health and human needs. More health care professionals need to take their knowledge to their state or national capital. Nurses have the education, experience, skills, and first-hand knowledge of health care and related issues to be successful in the legislative area.

Summary

Health care professionals must always be attuned to the ever-changing, and at times complex and burdensome, legalities that inundate the health care industry. Knowledge of legal issues, laws, regulations, and agencies at the local, state, and federal levels is a must, not only for themselves, but also for the good of their clients, clients' families, communities, and disciplines.

Nurses, while attending to their own practice issues, must advocate for their clients, especially in the areas of client rights, confidentiality, advance directives, and the unfortunate problems of client abuse and neglect. Nurses, by virtue of their education, experience, service, and social awareness are excellent candidates for board appointments and elected offices.

References

American Nurses Association. (1999). *Scope and standards of home health nursing practice.* Washington, DC: American Nurses Publishing.

Brent, N. J. (2001). *Nurses and the law* (2nd ed.). Philadelphia: Saunders.

Center for Medicare and Medicaid Services (August 8, 2005). *Guidance to surveyors: Home health agencies.*
   http://new.cms.hhs.gov/manuals/downloads/som107ap_b_hha.pdf

Christy, T. E. (1969). Portrait of a leader: Lavinia Lloyd Dock. *Nursing Outlook, 17*(6), 72–75.

Dailey, M., & Newfield, J. (2005). Legal issues in home care: Current trends, risk-reduction strategies, and opportunities for improvement. *Home Health Care Management & Practice, 17*(2), 93–100.

Des Jardin, K. E. (2001a). Political involvement in nursing—education and empowerment. *AORN Journal, 74*(4), 467–471, 473–479, 481–482.

Des Jardin, K. E. (2001b). Political involvement in nursing—politics, ethics, and strategic action. *AORN Journal, 74*(5), 613–615, 617–618, 621–626.

Duffy, B. (2001). Core curriculum for home health care nursing, (Section IV: Trends, issues, and research: Legal issues). Washington, DC: National Association for Home Care.

Guido, G. W. (2006). *Legal and ethical issues in nursing* (4th ed.). Upper Saddle River, NJ: Prentice-Hall.

Joint Commission on Accreditation of Healthcare Organizations (JCAHO). (2004). *Facts about the JCAHO*. Retrieved January 26, 2004, from
http://www.jcaho.org/about+us/index.htm

National Center on Elder Abuse. (1997). *Trends in elder abuse in domestic settings*. Retrieved June 20, 2004, from
http://www.elderabusecenter.org

Newfield, J. S. (2005). Current legal issues in providing wound care in the home. *Home Health Care Management & Practice, 17*(3), 233–242.

Pozgar, G. D. (2001). *Legal aspects of health care administration* (8th ed.). Gaithersburg, MD: Aspen.

Ramsey, G., & Mitty, E. (2003). Advance directives: Protecting patient's rights. In M. Mezey, T. Fulmer, & I. Abraham (Eds.), *Geriatric nursing protocols for best practice* (pp. 265–287). New York: Springer.

Rouse, F. (1991). Clients, providers, and the client self-determination act. *Hastings Center Report, 21*(1), S2–S3.

Russo, H. (2001). Window of opportunity for home care nurses: Telehealth technologies. *Online Journal of Issues in Nursing, 16*(3). Retrieved September 30, 2005, from
http://www.nursingworld.org/ojin/topic16/tpc16_4.htm

Stoker, J. (2003). Ten ways you can make a difference. *Home Healthcare Nurse, 21*(6), 382–383.

Tsai, C., & Starren, J. (2001). Patient participation in electronic medical records. *Journal of the American Medical Association, 285*(13), 1765.

Chapter 9

Ethics in Home Care and Hospice

Janie Butts, RN, DSN
Karen Rich, RN, PhD

Key Terms

Bioethics	Morality	Nursing Ethics
Ethics		

W hen considering ethics in home care and hospice, nurses might first question how home care and hospice ethics differs from ethics in other health care settings. There are moral considerations that are prominent in home care and hospice settings, but the important foundation of ethics is consistent across nursing practice areas. Although it is important to address various health care setting–specific ethical issues, for nurses to become *moral*, they must not compartmentalize morality based on ethical issues and situations according to different areas of practice. A moral nurse is first a moral person. Therefore, this chapter is presented with that view as a basis.

One purpose of this chapter is to explain some of the basic definitions, concepts, and approaches that are included in the philosophy of ethics. The second aim is to present for reflection ethical issues that are relevant to home care and hospice nursing. Though most people are influenced by societal norms and their culture, ethics is ultimately a personal matter, and deciding and acting according to what is good must be determined by each individual.

Nurses, in addition to their personal ethics, have professional codes of ethics to guide them in their ethical behavior and actions.

Overview of Ethics and Morality

Ethics is a branch of philosophy that is involved with proposing, analyzing, and describing how humans ought to be and act. **Morality** is how people actually do behave. Though many people define ethics and morality differently, the terms are frequently used interchangeably. When distinctions are made, they are usually in regard to the methodological nature of ethics as opposed to the more descriptive nature of morality. The meaning of right and wrong and the meaning and use of moral concepts, such as *good,* are examined in the field of philosophical ethics. Various moral theories, such as deontology and utilitarianism, have been developed by philosophers as a justification for resolving ethical situations. However, in this pluralistic society it can be argued that there cannot be one overriding theory, and there is no completely objective way to refute this argument. Because ethics is a branch of philosophy, it is approached differently than how one approaches science. Most ethicists, particularly those who are not objectivists, maintain that there is something elusive about finding the *truth* in relation to moral behavior.

Ethics can be divided into theoretical and applied ethics. Theoretical ethics is used to evaluate the consistency and foundation of ethical systems, whereas applied ethics involves the use of theories to guide practical behavior (Brannigan & Boss, 2001).

Another way ethics can be divided is according to the subject matter addressed. Normative ethics constitutes guidelines formed by the consensus of some group or community that governs moral behavior, such as the American Nurses Association (ANA) *Code of Ethics for Nurses,* originally created in 1926 (Viens, 1989). Ethical analysis of the use and meaning of moral concepts and moral statements forms the subject matter of meta-ethics. For example, meta-ethicists are interested in analyzing hard-to-define concepts such as the concept of *good* and statements that conflate a fact versus a value. Descriptive ethics involves the study of behaviors and belief systems. A nurse is doing descriptive ethics when conducting an observational study that generates data describing the moral behaviors and beliefs of nurses who work with vulnerable elderly clients in home care settings. If there is a possibility that ethics could be labeled as scientific, it is descriptive ethics that most closely meets scientific criteria.

Ethical issues that are specific to the field of health care are referred to as **bioethics.** The evolution of bioethics occurred primarily over a 40-year period from about 1947 to 1987 (Jonsen, 1998). The genesis of bioethics at that time was a result of the prosecution at the Nuremburg Trials of Nazi physicians who conducted inhumane experiments on Nazi prisoners during World War II. These war crimes served as the impetus for protecting human subjects during medical, social, and psychological research; these guidelines have continued to become more stringent over the years.

During the 1950s and 1960s, technological advancements in the areas of vaccination, transplantation, and life support pushed bioethical issues into the forefront of the human sciences. Human science professionals began to be asked crucial questions such as "Who should live?," "Who should die?," and "Who should decide?" (Jonsen, 1998, p. 11). Ironically, as society continues to search for solutions to life and death issues 50 years later, these same questions remain unanswered.

Ethical issues as they are particularly viewed and experienced by nurses are within a field of study apart from the application of ethics to other health care professionals, such as physicians. Bioethics and nursing ethics are not synonymous terms. However, because nurses are health care professionals, **nursing ethics** falls under the broad umbrella of bioethics, and nurses need to be well versed in this broad philosophical area. Nursing ethics specifically refers to proposing, analyzing, and describing ways that nurses ought to be and act regarding bioethical issues and nurses' everyday work. Nurses' relationships, including nurse-client, nurse-caregiver, nurse-family, nurse-significant other, nurse-nurse, and nurse-physician relationships, are important in the field of nursing ethics. Often, nurses are the connecting presence in health care relationships. This connecting presence presents an awe-inspiring ethical responsibility for nurses.

Virtue and Communitarian Ethics

Although there are many varying theories of ethics, virtue ethics and a communitarian approach seem to be at the center of a revival of tradition in ethics. These systems of ethics have a particular relevance for nursing because issues of character and relationships are inherently connected to professional nursing practice. Virtue ethics and a communitarian approach to ethics can be viewed separately, but some ethicists have drawn critical links between these two approaches (Blum, 1994; MacIntyre, 1984; Rich & Butts, 2005; Volbrecht, 2002).

Communitarian Ethics

According to Alasdair MacIntyre (1984), a virtue ethicist, communitarianism has its roots in the society of ancient Greek city-states. Communitarians place a value on the common good of communities, social goals, cooperative virtues, and tradition in practices (Beauchamp & Childress, 2001). In a communitarian ethical system, people are thought of as social beings with connected life stories or narratives. The fact that home care and hospice nurses practice nursing in their *community* does not mean that home care and hospice nurses are automatically communitarians in terms of its ethical meaning. Communitarian ethics is a philosophy of practice.

A fundamental basis of communitarian ethics is that it represents a reaction against the individualism popularized in Enlightenment-era philosophy. Wildes (2000) contended that, in bioethics, people must start from a point of community rather than from individuals. Because individuals cannot be separated from their communities, just as autonomous beings do not exist in isolation, communitarians view morality as an integral part of life within the community. Overriding communal goods and needs are prominent in communitarian ethics, and individual rights and needs are somewhat diminished.

Access to basic health care for all members of the community is an example of a common good. For all community members to have access to health care, other members of the community may have to make difficult sacrifices, such as paying higher taxes or relinquishing other services. When nurses pause and reflect on some community members' lack of access to needed home care and hospice services, nurses may decide that support for homebound and dying patients is not necessarily viewed as a common good. Communitarian ethics in nursing includes nurses' participation in changing public policy so that all members of the world community have access to basic health care.

Virtue Ethics

Virtue ethics, like communitarian ethics, has a long history with roots in ancient Greece since the time of Plato and Aristotle (Taylor, 2002). Plato and Aristotle were not really concerned with right and wrong in ways similar to how people think of these terms today. Aristotle was more concerned with *human excellence,* that is, the traits that are needed to help people best fulfill their human potential. Human excellence in Aristotle's idealized society was associated with a particular conception of friendship and the good life. This good life was closely tied to the political culture of the times. When the ancient Greeks considered right and wrong, it was usually in terms of the customs of the culture or the community. Individual excellence, or virtue, situated within the community and focused on the community's common good was a central ethical concern.

As opposed to emphasizing one's duty or the consequences of actions, virtue ethics is focused on the goodness or excellence of one's character. Rather than asking "What should I do?" a virtuous person asks "What sort of person should I become?" (Pojman, 2004, p. 388). Character is an overall balance of person's good (virtuous or excellent) traits weighed against their vices (undesirable traits). For example, a habitually truthful person has the character trait of honesty, even though someone who is habitually honest might occasionally tell a lie. All in all, however, one can rely on an honest person to value honesty. A virtuous person can be trusted to act virtuously in a preponderance of situations. Since the time of Plato and Aristotle, virtue ethicists have proposed that living a virtuous life, that is, being the way a virtuous person would be, leads to the highest form of living. Being virtuous has the ultimate effect of something akin to an enduring state of well-being or human flourishing.

Virtue ethics is especially relevant to home care and hospice nursing. In home care and hospice settings, nurses usually do not have direct on-site supervision during client care. In fact, the freedom and flexibility afforded in a home setting that allows for forms of autonomous nursing practice is what many nurses find appealing in regard to the practice setting. Enforcing ethical *rules* is often difficult in home care; clients and clinical managers generally rely on the *character* of the home care or hospice nurse to assure that quality and ethical care is provided.

The lack of direct observation by supervisors in home care and hospice settings leaves clients and agencies dependent on the good character of their nurses. Clients and supervisors to some extent must depend on a nurse's good character to provide the motivation to fulfill the directives of the *Code of Ethics for Nurses with Interpretive Statements* (ANA, 2001) that "the nurse's primary commitment is to the patient" (p. 9). Virtues are cultivated through habitually being and acting in ways that a person with good character would be and act. For example, if home care and hospice nurses habitually complete the full day's work for which they are paid, they are cultivating the virtue of honesty. Nurses might just as easily choose to cultivate the habit or vice of dishonesty by skimping on the time that they spend with clients and instead, for example, regularly do personal shopping during the hours that they are paid to care for clients.

The word *choose* in the last sentence of the preceding paragraph is a key word in terms of ethics. Most ethical situations for home care and hospice nurses are not the big bioethical issues that one often hears about on the news. Rather, nursing ethics is found in the day-to-day work of these nurses. Nurses have many opportunities to either choose virtuous behavior or to take an alternate, usually easier, path toward cultivating vices. In evaluating their virtues and values, home care and hospice nurses might ask themselves questions such as:

- Am I fully present and empathetic when I visit a client, or am I often thinking about what I want to do when I am finished with my workday?
- Do I provide clients with information such as test results, new physician's orders, and expected visit times to alleviate their anxiety, or am I too wrapped up in my own life to think about what might help my clients' emotional health?

A few of the many virtues that are important to home care and hospice nurses will be addressed in the following sections.

Truthfulness   Nurses may be surprised to realize how often deception enters into their practice. How often do nurses become rote with documentation? If client care documentation is not completely based on fact, it is deceptive. How often do nurses use self-deception to convince themselves that, because they are busy or they have other priorities, careless documentation is justified rather than being attentive to meticulous detail and narrative consistency? It is deceptive when home care nurses, who are paid according to the number of home visits they conduct, err on the side of describing their clients' conditions as more serious than they really are in order to keep the clients active with the agency and to increase the nurses' pay. Do nurses sometimes deceive themselves into thinking that they do not have time to spend with clients, such as a person experiencing death anxiety, who needs their compassionate presence?

Though truthfulness or veracity is a critical virtue for home care and hospice nursing, nurses working in these areas are often confronted with a dilemma about whether or not honest communication is the most compassionate action with clients. Ruddick (1999) proposed that a principle of hope-giving would be a valuable addition to traditional Western bioethical principles. The principle of autonomy has thrown hope-giving into a negative light because autonomy requires that persons be fully informed to self-direct their treatment.

It is not ethical for nurses to make a practice of lying to patients, but nurses must not respond too quickly without considered thought to questions from clients that are important in terms of their potential psychological impact. There is no algorithm to use to guide nurses in how to sensitively respond to questions from clients and their families. Sensitive and humanistic communication requires good judgment and a mature moral conscience. Strauss (2001) proposed helpful guidelines to use when visiting people with Alzheimer's disease, but her recommendations have wider applications for communicating with home care and hospice clients.

When nurses are asked questions about factual information, they may know the answer or need to obtain information to formulate an answer. However, sometimes nurses are asked questions that require answers that clients and families may not understand or may not really want to hear, such as questions about a client's prognosis. In these situations, nurses must be guided by their good judgment, their character, and their ethically educated intuition. There are no clear rules for communicating sensitively yet ethically. Strauss (2001) suggested "if you can't give a truthful answer that is believable, or acceptable or not hurtful at the cognitive level, then tell an emotional truth" (p. 14). Questions that are posed at the emotional as opposed to the cognitive level are questions that let nurses know that clients and families are "confused, depressed, scared, frustrated, or angry, or a combination of these feelings" (p. 15). Answering with an emotional truth involves acknowledging or validating the questioner's feelings without including blatant information that might be emotionally and unnecessarily hurtful.

Ruddick proposed, however, that though "deceptive hope may sometimes serve rather than subvert autonomy," health care professionals must not forget that "deception often separates patients and family in ways harmful to both" (p. 356). This separation can occur when deception is used by family members to keep unpleasant information from sick and dying loved ones. In trying to maintain hope, families can act in ways that thwart a loved one's peaceful death. Thus, compassionate deception must be used very judiciously and with careful forethought. In actuality, compassionate deception rarely would be considered virtuous behavior.

Compassion   Provision I of the *Code of Ethics for Nurses with Interpretive Statements* (ANA, 2001) states that "the nurse, in all professional relationships, practices with compassion" (p. 7). The virtue of compassion is a virtue that transcends cultural and philosophical boundaries. The traditional Buddhist conception of compassion is the desire to separate others from suffering. Buddhists believe that compassion can be developed to the point that its scope becomes unconditional, undifferentiated, and universal. It can extend toward all sentient beings, even to those who would harm us. The ultimate level in attainment of a compassion that is entirely dedicated to helping others overcome their suffering and the causes of their suffering is called *great compassion,* or *nying je chenmo.* Though attainment of this level of compassion is difficult, aspirations toward it can have a significant impact on one's outlook (Dalai Lama, 1999).

The Dalai Lama (1999) proposed that compassion is relevant to every area of life, including the workplace. When compassion is lacking and people ignore the impact of their actions on the well-being of others, their actions can sometimes become destructive and harmful. Frequently, clients in home care, and particularly hospice, settings are suffering physically, psychologically, and spiritually. The actions of nurses either may help to compassionately alleviate these clients' suffering, even in very small and incremental ways, or increase their suffering through a condescending pity or leave clients to feel isolated.

Just as Travelbee (1964) noted in her work with nurses, the Dalai Lama (1999) also mentioned that those people in the caring professions, including health care, might complain that feelings of compassion exhaust them in their work, causing them to feel emotionally burdened and physically fatigued. This compassion exhaustion can happen in any nursing job, but it may be particularly relevant for home care and hospice nurses who see the same long-term and chronic clients who do not significantly improve with medical treatments and nursing interventions. The Dalai Lama agreed that a continuous exposure to suffering, along with feeling that one's work is not appreciated, could prompt feelings of despair and helplessness among workers. These negative feelings, however, do not necessarily have to occur.

The cultivation of compassion requires a commitment to habits of acting compassionately. There are meditative practices that people, including nurses, can undertake to cultivate and enhance their levels of compassion, practices that do not increase one's exhaustion when done with single-minded concentration. One such example of a practice that can be used during client care is to meditate on exchanging oneself for another, which means that nurses must think about how they would feel and what they would want if they were the client. Using this meditation practice does not mean that nurses should act as if clients want the identical treatments that the nurses might desire. However, nurses can be fairly sure that most clients want to know that nurses care about them and that they want their nurses to attentively listen to them. This practice can be powerful for nurses in cultivating compassion.

Moral Courage   Moral courage is exhibited when a nurse can put fear aside to do the right thing and move forward. One must come to a testing point, that is, a "place where living according to moral principles may require us to put our comfort, possessions, relationships and careers at risk" in order for moral courage to be displayed (Josephson, 2002, p. 3).

Nurses may exhibit physical courage with brave acts from time to time, such as in responding to the September 11th disaster. However, everyday moral courage, sometimes more rare than physical courage, may be the greatest indicator of character (Josephson, 2002, p. 5). Moral courage is an everyday choice that nurses must make (Edmonds, 2001). Those nurses with poorly developed moral character sometimes make choices that are not optimal or ethical, such as self-serving types of choices.

Courage, or fortitude, from Plato's perspective is one of the four cardinal virtues—*cardinal* in Latin means *hinge,* which means that all other virtues *hinge* on the cardinal virtues (Kreeft, 1986). Some people believe that in order to do the right action, a person needs the highest sort of courage. In fact, Kreeft (1986) stated that the virtue of courage is so pivotal that if persons are not courageous, they will never overcome the difficulties of practicing any other virtue to its optimal level.

Home care and hospice nurses will face moral dilemmas and will be required to make difficult moral choices, such as whether or not to report a co-worker or an agency through appropriate channels when unethical practices are noticed. Nurses are directed in the *Code of Ethics for Nurses with Interpretive Statements* (ANA, 2001) to protect patients and the public from impaired practice of other workers. Virtuous nurses will be placed in positions of having to choose either to do the right thing at the right time and place even when these actions seem unpopular, difficult, beyond the call of duty, or just too much trouble; or to choose to act in ways that require fewer demands. Nurses sometimes must go the extra mile to do what is right, or what is virtuous, just for the sake of doing what is right.

Frequently, home care and hospice nurses can expect to meet resistance and be ridiculed when they make a moral choice to do the right thing despite efforts by others to persuade them otherwise. An example would be when a nurse has the perception that a physician is not adequately managing a dying client's cancer pain. A display of moral courage would be found in the nurse's not accepting the "brush-off" or harsh criticism from the physician who does not want to deal with the client's pain or who is just not knowledgeable enough about good pain management. Cultivating courage is worth the hardship that it entails because moral courage is a noble virtue.

Equanimity   The virtue of equanimity or even-mindedness points to the wisdom of equality and nondiscrimination, or the ability for people to see others as equal and to be impartial (Gunaratana, 2002; Salzberg, 2002). To abandon discrimination means to become "one" with the other, to put oneself "into the other person's skin" to the point that "there is no 'self' and no 'other'" (Thich Nhat Hanh, 1998, p. 175).

Equanimity is a serene state that must be cultivated so that a person develops an acceptance of life's imperfections (Salzberg, 2002). Developing the strength of equanimity requires that individuals understand that they cannot control the uncontrollable, such as events like the weather, and in the case of hospice nurses, for instance, death because of terminal disease.

When a very busy home care nurse can remain calm and balanced despite experiencing many external demands by physicians, agency personnel, clients, and families, the home care nurse exhibits or possesses the virtue of *equanimity*. In the following example, equanimity is highlighted. In the midst of a very hectic day, a nurse evaluates a client with only slightly worse breath sounds than usual. Even still, the nurse's intuition is that the client does not look quite right. Meanwhile, the nurse persists in calmness, calls the physician, and remains with the client, though she is concerned about her horrendous work schedule. The inner calmness of the nurse translates outwardly to the client, family, and physician as a balanced and even demeanor. When working toward equanimity, nurses develop personal responsibility, confidence in their actions, tough resilience, and a calm balanced state of mind that is not dependent on external situations.

Just Generosity   MacIntyre (1999) focused on an all-inclusive virtue of giving and receiving, *just generosity,* which is characterized by a type of charity. The virtue of just generosity is similar to a Lakota Indian expression that includes both elements of *justice* and *generosity, wancantognaka.* The term just generosity, as described by a Lakota Indian, Lydia Whirlwind Soldier (1996), "names a generosity that I owe to all those others who also owe it to me" (p. 11). There is no English word that represents these combined virtues.

Generosity is very powerful when people give freely to others without an attachment to any expectation in return. Salzberg (2002) added: "As we cultivate it [generosity], our heart will stop sticking to things" (p. 162). When generosity occurs in a spirit of non-attachment, just generosity has occurred.

Most people become needy and dependent on others at some point in their lives. Generous care for people who cannot care for themselves dates back as far as can be remembered in Eastern and Western cultures. Nurses may experience moral suffering when they see clients who they believe are in need of home care services but who must be denied care because of how regulatory rules are applied. Sometimes the rules that determine access to care within our health care system seem to be neither just nor generous.

With these constraints in mind, moral suffering can occur when nurses are the people who are actually in a position to decide whether or not to admit clients to a home care agency and to discharge clients who they believe may still need custodial care but not skilled care. In instances of client need when rules and regulations do not allow for covered services, nurses must be compassionate in facilitating as much support as possible for clients and families. Nurses who exhibit the virtue of just generosity will maintain a communitarian perspective of valuing networks of giving and receiving and connecting clients to these networks. Because of this valuing process, nurses may generously give their time toward aligning clients with helpful community resources.

Ron Sider (1999) elaborated on the importance of a healthy and flourishing civil society. Because human beings are social beings and made for communal living, people must be nurtured in warm, intimate, and wholesome environments within a community. In order to achieve healthy and optimal functioning, individuals need personal face-to-face relationships that provide just generosity. Sider (1999) developed a just generosity framework in which he stated: "Society should care—in a generous, compassionate way that strengthens dignity and respect—for those who cannot care for themselves" (p. 94).

Whether working in home care, hospice, hospitals, or clinics, nurses are advocates for their clients and are visionary and proactive leaders in health care. From the broader perspective of being responsible citizens, nurses with highly developed moral character make a difference in the community. The virtue of just generosity can be fulfilled through grassroots leadership activities in unity with the social networks in the community. Oftentimes, nurses are advocates for shaping public policy that will help those people who are disadvantaged and poor, need special health care, and have other unmet civil societal needs.

Moral Agency

Moral agency in ethics refers to a person's ability to make deliberate choices and take deliberate action in regard to moral behavior. Arguments in determining moral agency primarily result from debates about the client's mental competency in regard to making decisions. The issue is most often referred to in terms of whether or not a client is autonomous. However, other issues, such as attributions of inherent value and human vulnerability and dependence, are also related to moral agency. The issues in this section concerning moral agency overlap in content; however, to consider similar concepts and principles from various perspectives facilitates a broader understanding.

Autonomy

Autonomy in bioethics implies that persons are rational and capable of making their own medical decisions. Being one of the four principles of bioethics, along with beneficence, nonmaleficence, and justice, autonomy is an important concept in health care today. Allowing clients to freely make decisions regarding their health care is essential. Paternalism occurs when health care professionals make choices for a client "in the best interest of the client" or "for the client's own good." Over the years, medical personnel often exhibited paternalistic behavior, which eventually led to a backlash of elevated interest in respecting or protecting a client's autonomy.

As a communitarian, Hester (2001) is an ethicist who has proposed that healing requires communal involvement. When autonomy becomes the all-important focus in health care, communal involvement is often sidelined. In fact, Agich (2003) proposed that a societal overemphasis on autonomy in regard to elders creates ambivalence toward those people who are aged and dependent. Clients in home care and hospice need nursing, rehabilitation, and personal care because they have lost functional abilities, not because they lack autonomy. Suffering and need must be the primary focus of the client's care, not an overemphasis on rules and principles. When autonomy is viewed as constantly under threat, conflict and confusion often result. Consequently, older persons are not ennobled.

Agich (2003) highlighted an important point by stating that in an attempt to uphold the principle of autonomy, family caregivers should not be prevented from participating in decision making in regard to elderly clients. Family caregiver involvement in decisions does not necessarily imply that the elderly person is bound by those family decisions. In home care settings, caregivers, including nurses, are intimates, not strangers, to clients. Nurses can use practical reasoning skills in trying to discern whether capricious assumptions and prejudices are entering into families' decisions and health care events.

Vulnerability and Dependability

People often do not realize that there are alternative ways to address moral agency than solely from a primary position of the principle of autonomy. MacIntyre (1999) made an argument that humans need to acknowledge their animal nature along with their vulnerability and dependence if human well-being is to occur. For nurses and health care communities to flourish, the inherent value of each person must be supported.

MacIntyre (1999) proposed that our human nature cannot be separated from our animal nature, and advocated that this association must be acknowledged if we are to realize and benefit from knowing that we are all vulnerable and dependent during various points in our lives. As people grow from childhood to adulthood they normally progress from vulnerability and dependence to become persons capable of independent practical reasoning.

When vulnerability and dependence are discussed in terms of ethics, the focus is in regard to the need for stronger people to bestow their virtues on vulnerable and dependent people with giving flowing only in one direction, that is, toward the vulnerable (MacIntyre, 1999). On the other hand, just generosity involves an unconditional giving and receiving flowing in both directions. Those who are currently not in a position of dependence, like nurses, realize that "there but for the grace of God go I" and acknowledge their human vulnerability. In thinking this way, the nurse can become open to learning through the narrative of clients' stories.

Competence

Questions of competence are associated most often with mentally disabled people, cognitively impaired elderly people, and children (Stanley, Sieber, & Melton, 2003, p. 398). Competence is closely tied to formal situations that legally require informed consent. Though clients in home care settings generally do not undergo the same level of invasive procedures that are rendered in an acute care setting, assessing clients' competence remains an important ethical consideration. With children, most nurses realize the ethical and legal implications of obtaining consent from parents or legal guardians. For mentally disabled and cognitively impaired clients, however, determining competence is not always easy.

Although there are a number of different perspectives about how to determine clients' competence, one method of determining competence is unique because it includes a range of *inabilities* that someone who is incompetent would exhibit (Beauchamp & Childress, 2001). The standards begin by requiring the least ability that indicates competence and move toward those activities that require higher ability. The standards are:

1. Inability to express or communicate a preference or choice.
2. Inability to understand one's situation and its consequences.
3. Inability to understand relevant information.
4. Inability to give a reason.
5. Inability to give a rational reason (although some supporting reasons may be given).
6. Inability to give risk/benefit-related reasons (although some rational supporting reasons may be given).
7. Inability to reach a reasonable decision (as judged, for example, by a reasonable person standard). (p. 73.)

Sometimes nurses may too quickly assume that vulnerable and dependent clients are incompetent and do not need to be brought into caregiving or other life decisions that involve them. An example might be something as simple as a nurse's not asking for a client's preference regarding how a bath is to be given, to something as serious as a nurse assisting or supporting a family member in taking legal control of an elderly, but still competent, client's material assets.

Dignity and Dementia

Oftentimes nurses in a home care setting are charged with caring for clients with dementia. Kitwood (1997) proposed that because of our cultural development, society and health care communities have been responsible for treating demented persons as the "new outcasts of society" (p. 44). According to Jenkins and Price (1996), the loss experienced by persons with dementia can be likened to a loss of personhood.

People who become accustomed to a demented person's decline often begin treating the demented person as less than a person (Moody, 1992). Even though persons with dementia seem to fade bit by bit from the person that they once seemed to be, they may still be aware of their feelings. Conceivably, an extreme sense of vulnerability can occur during the early and middle stages of a progressive dementia when cognitive ability is still present in terms of awareness of personhood and connectedness to the environment and to others.

Provision 1.1 of the *Code of Ethics for Nurses with Interpretive Statements* (ANA, 2001) is "respect for human dignity" (p. 7). Risk of losing the sense of dignity is high for clients with dementia because of the awareness that these persons have in regard to how others view them, again, making them what Kitwood (1997) referred to as outcasts. When caregivers are intently focused on making ethical decisions regarding care of persons with dementia, the importance of daily human interactions and relatedness, the place where real dignity is or is not attributed, often gets lost (Moody, 1992).

Nurses can compassionately try to alleviate the suffering experienced by persons with dementia and their families. The equanimity and care exhibited by the nurse can be very valuable in serving as an example of a disposition in caregiving that anxious and frustrated family caregivers can try to emulate. Extending care and kindness can go a long way toward fostering a sense of dignity, which a demented person may be in the process of losing. Nurses also can practice gentle communication when giving care to persons with dementia. Gentle words and actions toward demented clients promote calmness, whereas harsh and loud words provoke fear and anxiousness.

End of Life

Frequently clients receiving home care services are seriously ill and functionally disabled and will likely receive hospice care as they approach the end of their lives. End-of-life care can be confusing and morally stressful for nurses, clients, and family caregivers. Though end-of-life care is an everyday part of hospice situations, it often presents an ethical minefield for nurses when clients explore or choose options that are controversial according to the norms of societal thinking.

Death comes to everyone, and almost no one wants to prolong suffering. Sometimes the circumstances surrounding the death and dying experience bring emotional, financial, and social burdens upon families and clients in ways that promote euthanasia's strong appeal (Munson, 2004). Euthanasia, meaning "good death" in Greek or what has come to mean "easy death," is divided into two basic forms: active, which is to take a definitive action, such as administering a lethal injection of a medication; and passive, which means to allow death to occur without intervention (p. 690).

Technology has prompted mass scrutiny about death and has caused society to be skeptical about the traditional way that death has been defined in the past. High technology and the focus on the person's autonomy have given society a greater variety of choices concerning end-of-life decisions, such as withholding or withdrawing life support, voluntary stopping of eating and drinking (VSED), terminal sedation (TS), rational suicide, and physician-assisted suicide (PAS).

Home care and hospice nurses must participate in a collaborative decision-making process with other health team members, as well as with families and clients, when decisions about end-of-life issues are made (Ladd, Pasquerella, & Smith, 2002). Listening to concerns raised by family members or clients, asking the type of questions that will help families and clients to explore their own feelings and beliefs, and focusing on the individual needs of families and clients, such as psychiatric consultation, are the type of responsible and ethical roles that home care and hospice nurses will fulfill.

Death Anxiety

Death anxiety may be an overlooked source of suffering for clients, families, and even nurses. Death anxiety becomes a moral issue when one considers that those who experience it frequently become detached from these feelings. Therefore, relationships may suffer. The underlying pervasiveness of death anxiety that has affected humans since the beginning of time is highlighted in the Latin proverb "the fear of death is worse than death," as cited by H. L. Mencken (1942, p. 267). In a narrative sense, an individual may believe that death is how the story ends. Perhaps existential philosophers have presented it best in identifying death anxiety as one of the most fundamental existential issues that all people face.

According to Yalom (1980), the fear of death is a primitive source of anxiety and is one of the main sources of psychological disorders. Existential philosophers believe that death anxiety is often denied, sublimated, or converted in attempts to maintain the balance in life that most people seek but often cannot obtain.

Death anxiety cannot be recognized unless the nurse uses compassionate listening to identify the client's fear of death, which is being written "between the lines." Being a compassionate nurse involves wanting to separate the client from suffering. Though it may not be feasible to completely resolve a client's death anxiety, acting from compassion would include acting from insight into how the fear of death and the realization of the impermanence of one's life enter into the context of a client's life story.

Death anxiety from the perspective of the client is an important issue. However, another issue, which is possibly more important in terms of its effect on client care, is nurses' experiences with their own death anxiety. A nurse who is experiencing death anxiety may become detached from clients in ways that are unfavorable to engaging in the narrative of moral care. Facing the often hard to identify effects of death anxiety can be a life-changing experience for nurses as well as for clients.

Withholding and Withdrawing Life Support

For home care and hospice nurses, the acts of withholding and withdrawing life support are some of the most challenging ethical issues that will be faced. Although in its *Code of Ethics for Nurses with Interpretive Statements* Provision 1.3 the ANA (2001) takes the position that nurses should never participate in intentional and active euthanasia, the ANA does encourage nurses to provide supportive and compassionate end-of-life care to clients.

Competent clients have a right to exercise their autonomy when deciding to accept or refuse any medical treatment. However, when competent clients choose their end-of-life care treatments, home care and hospice nurses must try to assure that decisions are free of coercion from other health care staff or from family members (Ladd, Pasquerella, & Smith, 2002). It is the responsibility of home care and hospice nurses, first, to educate their clients regarding their rights and options, and second, to support their clients in their decisions to refuse treatment.

When clients are mentally incompetent, the avenue for the client's self-determination is the advance directive. If an advance directive has not been completed, a surrogate decision-maker is used, usually a close family member. Sometimes, the courts will assign a surrogate or guardian. Often a family member has difficulty in "letting go" despite information received from the health team that treatment is futile.

Futile care refers to treatment that is of no physiological benefit for a terminally ill client (Beauchamp & Childress, 2001). It is essential that futility issues be discussed among family members, clients, and the health care team if at all possible. Home care and hospice nurses need to identify the client's surrogate decision-maker and then try to assure that a decision-making process is facilitated so that everyone has a chance to express feelings and concerns (Ladd, Pasquerella, & Smith, 2002).

Voluntarily Stopping Eating and Drinking

Voluntarily stopping nutrition in the form of eating and drinking is the prerogative of a client who has the mental capacity to choose to refuse food and fluids (Quill & Byock, 2000). Though some people consider the refusal of nutrition and hydration to be a form of suicide, other people believe that clients have the right to refuse these treatments. Those people who advocate this right of refusal sometimes view the prolongation of life in a terminal state to be meaningless and without value. Voluntarily stopping eating and drinking, or foregoing of life-sustaining therapy, cannot be ordered or directed by the physician, which is generally advantageous for clients.

When a client decides to refuse nutrition, however, the support of home care and hospice nurses, physicians, and family members is essential. The ANA takes the position that, because competent clients have the right to choose the acceptance or refusal of food and fluid, nurses must continue to provide support, promote dignity, and provide high-quality care (ANA, 1992). Home care and hospice nurses must respect the client's right to make the decision to forego life-sustaining therapy, which may include food and fluids.

Rule of Double Effect

The rule of double effect, first developed by the Catholic Church in the Middle Ages, allows the use of high doses of pain medication to lessen the intractable pain of terminally ill persons even if death is precipitated by administration of the medication (Quill, 2001). The primary determination in using this rule is that the harmful effect (death) is not the *intended* effect, although the harmful effect may be a *foreseen* event. Quill listed the key elements of the rule as:

1. The act must be good or at least morally neutral.
2. The agent must intend the good effect and not the evil effect (which may be "foreseen" but not intended).
3. The evil effect must not be the means to the good effect.
4. There must be a "proportionally grave reason" to risk the evil effect. (p. 167.)

Provision 1.3 of the *Code of Ethics for Nurses with Interpretive Statements* (ANA, 2001) supports nurses in acting to relieve dying clients' pain "even when those interventions entail risks of hastening death" (p. 8). However, the code is clearly consistent with the rule of double effect, in mandating that the act must never be deliberately undertaken to end a client's life even if nurses believe that they are acting compassionately.

Nurses who find themselves in situations where they are considering the rule of double effect as a factor in their client care, and who are uncomfortable with the ethical implications, need to discuss their concerns with their supervisors. It is natural for conscientious nurses to feel unsure when they are involved with such ethically laden situations, but obtaining guidance from the ANA code, ethicists, and trusted senior members of the health care team will help nurses to work through ethical dilemmas in client care.

Terminal Sedation

Terminal sedation (TS) is a legally permissible, but ethically controversial, action, although ethical consensus is growing in the direction of acceptance (Quill, 2001). According to Quill, "TS occurs when a suffering client is sedated to unconsciousness, usually through the ongoing administration of barbiturates or benzodiazepines. The client then dies of dehydration, starvation, or some other intervening complication, as all other life-sustaining interventions are withheld" (p. 181). After sedation is begun, the client may live days or weeks. Terminal sedation is used in situations in which a terminally ill client experiences extreme suffering and pain.

As with the rule of double effect, the intended effect in the administration of pain medication is to relieve suffering, not to intentionally cause death. Therefore, death is *foreseen* but not *intended,* which according to many people is a mere technicality in regard to the ethics of using terminal sedation. It is this ambiguous situation that seems similar to physician-assisted sedation that prevents ethical consensus in regard to terminal sedation.

Physician-Assisted Suicide

The controversy over physician-assisted suicide goes back to Greek and Roman times (Boyd, 2003). In 1994 in the state of Oregon, a Death with Dignity Act was passed, which permits terminally ill clients to obtain prescriptions to end their lives under certain safeguards in a humane and dignified manner. Oregon remains the only state in the United States where assisted suicide is legally practiced.

During a long 20-year dispute, active euthanasia was permitted under certain special guidelines in the Netherlands (Boyd, 2003). In February 2002, a Dutch law was passed permitting voluntary euthanasia and physician-assisted suicide. There is, however, a philosophical difference in the way that people in the Netherlands and the United States have discussed the issue of euthanasia. In the United States, debates about euthanasia have primarily focused only on physician-assisted suicide, whereas in the Netherlands debates have included a wider perspective on euthanasia.

In the United States, there has been everything from moral outrage to moral acceptance regarding physician-assisted suicide. Boyd (2003) emphasized that the public needs to be educated about legal and ethical options concerning end-of-life care and the consequences regarding any decision that is made. The Oregon Nurses Association has issued special guidelines for nurses related to the Death with Dignity Act (cited in Ladd, Pasquerella, & Smith, 2002).

In the guidelines, the Oregon Nurses Association confirmed the need for client support, comfort, and confidentiality. The Association also advised nurses in Oregon to explore options regarding end-of-life decisions and resources with their clients, to discuss reasons for the decision, to be present during the client's self-administration of the medications and during the client's death, and to be involved in policy development regarding home and community care. Explicitly, in Oregon the nurse may not inject or administer the medication that leads to death; breach confidentiality; make judgmental statements; subject others, including peers, to judgmental comments about the client; or abandon or refuse care to or safety measures for the client (Ladd, Pasquerella, & Smith, 2002).

In Oregon, one important point regarding the issue of physician-assisted suicide in a home care and hospice setting is the need for initiating a collaborative team approach. A team approach minimizes confusion and misunderstandings about communication regarding the wishes and desires of the client and family. Like terminal sedation, physician-assisted suicide provokes an uncertain moral state of affairs.

Rational Suicide

For terminally ill clients, the process of their trying to achieve a "good death" can be overwhelming. Debilitated or dying clients many times view suicide as an escape from life or an escape from a long and lingering wait permeated with pain and suffering. Suicide has been controversial for as long as the term has been known. However, as years have passed, there have been varied opinions of suicide—from social acceptance to social disapproval, depending on religious convictions, secular criminalization, and medicalization (Johnstone, 1999). Generally, nursing attitudes have been aligned with society's attitudes of rational suicide.

Rational suicide is defined as self-slaying that is characterized by reasoned choice and seems to make sense to other people. The issue of suicide, rational or not, is very relevant for nurses, because each year in the United States alone, 30,622 suicides are reported annually (Centers for Disease Control and Prevention, 2005).

No matter what is decided by rational, terminally ill clients about ending their lives, home care and hospice nurses need to inquire about clients' reasons for suicide decisions and explore possible alternatives without judgmental and coercive undertones. The moral issues for home care and hospice nurses surrounding rational suicide are very complex and require unique support and intervention for each and every client and family member; therefore, nurses are treading on uncertain moral ground.

Summary

Over the years, home care and hospice nursing has become more ethically complex as more intensive and highly technological treatments have become commonplace in the home, access to care has become more restricted, regulatory standards have become more complicated, and life expectancy has continued to increase. Consequently, nurses often find themselves feeling as if they are not on solid ground when trying to navigate through the daily aspects of client care. There are no easy algorithms or methods to sort out all ethical dilemmas; however, the good moral character of each nurse can remain consistent. A good nurse must first be a good person, and the virtues are a path to flourishing moral ground. A nurse can cultivate a strong moral character by making a conscious and habitual effort to read nursing literature about client care, by maintaining competency in practice, and by acting in virtuous ways such as displaying the virtues discussed in this chapter—truthfulness, moral courage, compassion, equanimity, and just generosity.

References

American Nurses Association. (2001). *Code of ethics for nurses with interpretive statements.* Washington, DC: ANA.

American Nurses Association. (1992). *Position statement: Foregoing nutrition and hydration.* Retrieved January 4, 2006, from
http://nursingworld.org/readroom/position/ethics/prtetnutr.htm

Agich, G.J. (2003). *Dependency and autonomy in old age: An ethical framework for long-term care* (2nd & rev. ed.). Cambridge, UK: Cambridge University Press.

Beauchamp, T. L., & Childress, J. F. (2001). *Principles of biomedical ethics* (5th ed.). New York: Oxford University Press.

Blum, L. A. (1994). *Moral perception and particularity.* New York: Cambridge University Press.

Boyd, A. D. (2003). *Physician-assisted suicide: For and against.* Retrieved January 2, 2006, from
http://www.amsa.org/bio/pas.cfm

Brannigan, M. C., & Boss, J.A. (2001). *Health care ethics in a diverse society.* Mountain View, CA: Mayfield Publishing Co.

Centers for Disease Control and Prevention. (2005, December 5). National Center for Disease Prevention and Control: Suicide Fact Sheet. Retrieved December 27, 2005, from
http://www.cdc.gov/ncipc/factsheets/suifacts.htm

Dalai Lama (1999). *Ethics for the new millennium.* New York: Riverhead Books.

Edmonds, B. (2001). Courage? LewRockwell.com. Retrieved January 4, 2006, from
http://www.lewrockwell.com/edmonds/edmonds60.html

Gunaratana, B. H. (2002). *Mindfulness: In plain English*. (Updated & expanded ed.). Boston: Wisdom Publications.

Hester, D. M. (2001). *Community as healing: Pragmatist ethics in medical encounters*. Lanham, MD: Rowman & Littlefield Publishers, Inc.

Jenkins, D., & Price, B. (1996). Dementia and personhood: A focus for care? *Journal of Advanced Nursing, 24*(1), 84-90.

Johnstone, M. J. (1999). *Bioethics: A nursing perspective* (3rd ed.). Sydney, Australia: Harcourt Saunders.

Jonsen, A. (1998). *The birth of bioethics*. New York: Oxford University Press.

Josephson, M. (2002, February 13). A few thoughts on moral courage. *Ethics Briefs*, 7(1). Retrieved January 6, 2006, from
http://ethics.jpl.nasa.gov/briefs/vol7is1/ethicsbites.html

Kitwood, T. (1997). *Dementia reconsidered: The person comes first*. Buckingham, UK: Open University Press.

Kreeft, P. (1986). Justice, wisdom, courage, & moderation: The four cardinal virtues. *Back to virtue* (Chap. 4, pp. 59-70). San Francisco: Ignatius Press. Retrieved January 5, 2006, from
http://www.catholiceducation.org/articles/religion/re0017.html

Ladd, R. E., Pasquerella, L., & Smith, S. (2002). *Ethical issues in home health care*. Springfield, IL: Charles C. Thomas.

MacIntyre, A. (1999). *Dependent rational animals: Why human beings need the virtues*. Chicago, IL: Open Court.

MacIntyre, A. (1984). *After virtue*. Notre Dame, IN: University of Notre Dame Press.

Mencken, H. L. (1942). *A new dictionary of quotations on historical principles from ancient and modern sources*. New York: Alfred A. Knopf.

Moody, H. R. (1992). *Ethics in an aging society*. Baltimore, MD: Johns Hopkins University Press.

Munson, R. (2004). *Intervention and reflection: Basic issues in medical ethics* (7th ed.). Sydney, Australia: Thomson Wadsworth.

Pojman, L. P. (2004). *The moral life: An introductory reader in ethics and literature*. New York: Oxford University Press.

Quill, T. E. (2001). *Caring for clients at the end of life: Facing an uncertain future together*. New York: Oxford University Press.

Quill, T. E., & Byock, I. R. (2000). Responding to intractable terminal suffering: The role of terminal sedation and voluntary refusal of food and fluids. (American College of Physicians— American Society of Internal Medicine.) *Annals of Internal Medicine, 132,* 408-414. Retrieved January 5, 2006, from
http://www.dyingwell.com/downloads/terminalsufferingannals00.pdf

Rich, K. L., & Butts, J. B. (2005). Values, relationships, and virtues. In J. B. Butts & K. L. Rich, *Nursing Ethics: Across the Curriculum and into Practice* (pp. 29-52). Boston: Jones and Bartlett Publishers.

Ruddick, W. (1999). Hope and deception. *Bioethics, 13*(3/4), 343-357.

Salzberg, S. (2002). *Lovingkindness: The revolutionary art of happiness.* Boston: Shambhala.

Sider, R. (1999). *Just generosity: A new vision for overcoming poverty in America.* Grand Rapids, MI: Baker Books.

Soldier, L. W. (1996). Wancantognaka: The continuing Lakota custom of generosity. *Tribal College Journal, 7*(3), 10-12.

Stanley, B., Sieber, J. E., & Melton, G. B. (2003). Empirical studies of ethical issues in research: A research agenda. In D. N. Bersoff (Ed.), *Ethical Conflicts in Psychology* (3rd ed., pp. 398-402). Washington, DC: American Psychological Association.

Strauss, C. J. (2001). *Talking to Alzheimer's.* Oakland, CA: New Harbinger Publications.

Taylor, R. (2002). *Virtue ethics: An introduction.* Amherst, NY: Prometheus Books.

Thich Nhat Hanh. (1998). *The heart of the Buddha's teaching: Transforming suffering into peace, joy, and liberation.* New York: Broadway Books.

Travelbee, J. (1964). What's wrong with sympathy? *The American Journal of Nursing,* January, 68-71.

Viens, D. C. (1989). A history of nursing's code of ethics. *Nursing Outlook, 37*(1), 45-49.

Volbrecht, R. M. (2002). *Nursing ethics: Communities in dialogue.* Upper Saddle River, NJ: Prentice-Hall.

Wildes, K. W. (2000). *Moral acquaintances: Methodology in bioethics.* Notre Dame, IN: University of Notre Dame Press.

Yalom, I. D. (1980). *Existential psychotherapy.* New York: Basic Books.

Chapter 10

Quality Improvement

Patsy Anderson, RN, DNS

Key Terms

Outcome	Performance Improvement	Quality
		Risk Adjustment

Home care nurses have many responsibilities, one of which is to provide quality client care in a cost-effective manner. This may sound easy, but the task is arduous. According to Barnum and Kerfoot (1995), many nurses lack the expertise to assess, understand, and achieve quality outcomes that promote quality cost-effective programs. The responsibility to assess quality is most often delegated to a group of professionals who understand performance-improvement strategies and techniques. Home care nurses are often not involved in quality assessment due to a lack of understanding of the processes needed to assure quality.

Quality

Health care experts have struggled for decades in an attempt to develop a single meaningful, acceptable definition of the quality of health care. There are now several commonly cited definitions, which differ in their emphasis on the quality of life, the service delivery, and the processes of care as components of quality.

A 1990 definition from the Institute of Medicine, which was arrived at after collecting and considering over 100 definitions of quality from the literature, appears often in discussions of the quality of medical care. The Institute of Medicine defined **quality** as "the degree to which health services for individuals and populations increase the likelihood that desired health outcomes is consistent with current professional knowledge" (Richardson & Corrigan, 2002, p. 1). This definition is important to home care nurses because it is currently the most cited and professionally recognized medical definition of quality health care. Quality, as defined by the Joint Commission, is:

> (a) a character, characteristic, or property of anything that makes it good or bad, commendable or reprehensible; thus the degree of excellence that a thing possesses; and
> (b) the totality of features and characteristics of a product or service that bear on its ability to satisfy. (JCAHO, 1996, p. 129).

According to the JC, an **outcome** in health care is "the cumulative effect at a defined point in time of performing one or more processes in the care of a client" (JCAHO, 1996, p.28). The Center for Medicare and Medicaid Services (2003) defines an outcome as "a change in client health status between two or more points in time."

Avedis Donabedian first suggested that there is more than one legitimate formulation of quality depending on the system of care and the nature and extent of responsibilities. He describes four main perspectives on quality: the health care professional perspective, the client perspective, the perspective of health care plans and organizations, and the purchaser perspective, all of which lead to different definitions of quality. Health care providers tend to view quality in terms of the attributes of care and the results of care, leading to definitions of quality that emphasize technical excellence and the characteristics of client/professional interaction (Donabedian, 1988).

Perspectives on Quality

The perspective from which quality is viewed defines its characteristics. Several viewpoints are now discussed.

- Clients tend to view quality in terms of their own preference and values, leading to definitions of quality that encompass satisfaction with care, as well as outcomes such as decreased morbidity, mortality, and improved functional status.
- Health care plans and organizations that deliver services tend to place greater emphasis on the general health of the enrolled or covered population and on the functioning of the organization. This perspective, which encompasses decisions to limit some care to assure essential services for all, acknowledges the reality of fixed resources.
- Purchasers, such as health care organizations, tend to be concerned about population-based measures of quality and organization performance. The purchaser perspective leads to a definition of quality that is similar to that of health care organizations. However, purchasers are concerned about the "value" of care, and this concern incorporates the price of care and the efficiency of the delivery of care.

Quality Improvement

The distinction between quality and performance measurement is not clear in the published literature. Performance measurement is the term usually applied when an organization is being assessed and when access, cost, and efficiency are being assessed as a component of quality.

Some people would say that quality improvement is in the eye of the beholder. This concept is known by many different names such as total quality management, quality assurance, continuous quality improvement, performance improvement, statistical quality control, and statistical process control. With quality improvement being called many names, it is no wonder that many nurses do not understand exactly what organizational leadership is talking about when the term quality improvement is discussed (JCAHO, 1993). Nurses who are engaged in quality/performance improvement have found that the process is very similar to the nursing process.

The public has just begun to recognize that despite the enormous achievements of American medicine and the American health care system, the quality of care in this country needs to be and can be improved. Recent reports from the Institute of Medicine dramatized the need for greater attention not only to potential problems with quality but also to the entire structure of the delivery system. The reports proposed several approaches to improving the quality of American health care; these approaches are based on control of overuse, misuse, and under use of drugs, devices and procedures (Richardson & Corrigan, 2002).

Quality Experts

Through the years, since quality, quality performance, and quality improvement have become topics of research and study, several students of the discipline have distinguished themselves to the point of being referred to as quality experts.

W. Edwards Deming   W. Edwards Deming has been described as a national folk hero in Japan due to his spectacular influence on the rise of Japanese industry after World War II, a rise that resulted in an unprecedented level of quality and productivity in Japan. Deming was trained as a physicist, obtaining a doctorate at Yale University in 1928. Due to his work at the United States Department of Agriculture (USDA) and his expertise in statistics, Deming was sent to Japan in 1946 by the War Department to study agricultural production and related problems. During his five trips to Japan, Deming was able to give the Japanese not only statistical theory but also an increasing level of confidence. Deming told the Japanese that by using his methods they could capture the world market in five years; instead, they accomplished it in four years (Walton, 1996).

Deming pursued a similar goal in the United States, but it took much longer for Americans to appreciate his teachings than it had for the Japanese. The United States did not recognize Deming as a guru in quality until Japanese competition awakened the business community. Deming emphasized the process over the product. He recognized that inspecting faults was costly in terms of inspection, reprocessing, and angry customers. Deming's approach to quality is encapsulated in his famous 14 points for management, which are summarized in Box 10-1 (Walton, 1996).

Joseph Juran   Joseph Juran was a statistician like Deming, who also contributed to Japanese management. Juran's definition of quality had two components: a product feature that meets customer needs and freedom from deficiencies or error rate. Juran founded the Juran Institute, a training institute for quality. He also promoted ideas relating to the integration

---

BOX 10-1 DEMING'S 14 POINTS OF QUALITY

Point 1: Create constancy of purpose toward improvement of product and service.

Point 2: Adopt the new philosophy.

Point 3: Cease dependence on inspection to achieve quality.

Point 4: End the practice of awarding business on the basis of price tag.

Point 5: Improve constantly and forever the system of production and service.

Point 6: Institute training on the job.

Point 7: Institute leadership.

Point 8: Drive out fear, so that everyone may work effectively for the company.

Point 9: Break down barriers between departments.

Point 10: Eliminate slogans, exhortations, and targets by the workforce.

Point 11: Eliminate numerical quotas and management by objective.

Point 12: Remove barriers to pride of workmanship.

Point 13: Institute a vigorous program of education and self-improvement.

Point 14: Put everyone in the organization to work to accomplish the transformation. (Deming, 1986.)

---

of quality improvement into corporate plans, quality as being fitness for purpose rather than conformance to specification, teamwork, delighting customers, and problem solving (Juran, 1989). In the early 1960s, a wave of leading corporations began to undertake mass deployment of quality tools. Previously, only small groups of quality control experts learned how to analyze work processes, reduce variation, and improve quality and cost (Juran 1989). Juran's definition appears in Box 10-2.

Juran also developed the Juran Trilogy, which identified three processes: quality planning, quality control, and quality improvement. Through these processes, managers could maintain and improve quality (Box 10-3).

Philip Cosby Philip Cosby developed a framework for total quality management that focused on zero defects. Zero defects was the performance standard applied to all measurement because Cosby believed that quality is measurable by the cost of nonconformance and must always be done right the first time (Cosby, 1979). Cosby began his quality experience as a line inspector for International Telephone and Telegraph and rose to corporate vice president. This allowed him to have a unique perspective on the evaluation of quality. Quality, according to Cosby, includes conformance to requirements, prevention, and measurement. His programs converge on stress behaviors, values, statistical techniques, and practice tools

BOX 10-2 JURAN'S DEFINITION OF QUALITY

Product Features That Meet Customer Needs
- Increase customer satisfaction.
- Make products saleable.
- Meet competition.
- Increase market share.
- Provide sales income.
- Secure premium prices.

Freedom from Deficiencies
- Reduce error rates.
- Reduce rework waste.
- Reduce field failure and warranty charges.
- Reduce inspection; test shortens time to new products on the market.
- Increase yields and capacity.
- Improve delivery performance. (Juran, 1989.)

BOX 10-3 JURAN'S TRILOGY

Quality Planning (building quality)
- Determine who the customers are.
- Determine the needs of the customers.
- Develop product features that respond to customers' needs.
- Develop processes able to produce the product features.
- Transfer the plans to the operating forces.

Quality Control (maintaining the status quo)
- Evaluate actual performance.
- Compare actual performance to goals.
- Take action on the differences.

Quality Improvement (significant improvement in operations)
- Establish the necessary infrastructure.
- Identify the specific improvement projects.
- Establish a team for each project.
- Provide the resources, motivation, and training for the teams.
- Teams diagnose the causes, establish or stimulate a remedy, and establish controls to hold the gains. (Juran, 1989.)

BOX 10-4 COSBY'S FOUR ABSOLUTES OF QUALITY

1. The definition of quality is conformance to requirements (do it right the first time).
   - Establish the requirements that employees are to meet.
   - Supply the wherewithal that the employees need in order to meet those requirements.
   - Spend time helping the employees meet those requirements.
2. The system of quality is prevention.
   - Prevention is improving the process so that errors or problems don't occur in the first place.
   - Avoid work arounds to solve problems.
   - Use statistical quality control methods.
3. The performance standard is zero defects.
   - Requirements must be met.
4. The measure of quality is the price of nonconformance.
   - Includes all the expenses involved in doing things wrong.
   (Cosby, 1995.)

(Cosby, 1984). Cosby became well known with the publication, in 1979, of his book *Quality Is Free.* Like Deming, Cosby emphasized the importance of systems knowledge and improvement, the drawbacks of inspection, and the need for statistical control. Cosby's Four Absolutes of Quality are given in Box 10-4.

Health Care's History of Quality

During the past several decades, hospitals were required by regulatory agencies, in particular the Joint Commission (JC), to comply with vague guidelines related to assuring quality. From 1953 through 1974, the JC's method of examining quality was limited to morbidity and mortality studies where specific cases for individual failures were cited and the individual was reprimanded. In 1975, the JC began to require formal audits of certain hospital services by examining specific objectives. However, the audits were isolated. In 1988, the JC implemented the accreditation of home care organizations using the same requirement for quality improvement as for hospitals (Capezio & Morehouse, 1993).

Performance Improvement

JC defined **performance improvement** as "the study and adaptation of functions and processes to increase the probability of achieving desired outcomes" (JCAHO, 1999, p. 164). This definition is applied to all health care accredited organizations including home care. The following sections describe the processes that can be used in home care organizations in the performance-improvement process. Performance improvement focuses on the processes that organizations use and their attempts to continuously improve the design of those processes.

Increasingly, external groups such as purchasers and payers of health care are demanding that health care organizations are able to satisfy their customers, contain costs, and have desirable outcomes. Consumers, an external group, are also much more interested in the performance of their health care providers than are internal groups. Organizations also have found that the use of performance- improvement processes can directly impact the care they provide. Performance improvement focuses on the processes that organizations use and their attempts to continuously improve the design of those processes (Friedman, 2000).

Performance-Improvement Methods   No matter how sophisticated or highly computerized an organization is, process improvement requires a systematic method. That method is one that ensures that improvement actions are based on sound data and analysis and that the actions result in the desired outcomes. There have been many such performance-improvement models developed.

Plan-Do-Check-Act   One of the most commonly used performance-improvement models is the Plan-Do-Check-Act (PDCA) model, also called the Shewhart cycle. This model was extensively used and taught by Deming. *Plan* refers to deciding how an improvement action will be tested and how data will be collected to determine what effect the action has. *Do* means to perform the test by implementing the action on a small scale. *Check* involves analyzing the effect of the action being tested. *Act* means fully implementing the action. This model is useful in planning, testing, assessing, and implementing an action to improve a process (McNeil, 2001). An alternate name for PDCA is Plan-Do-Study-Act, or PDSA.

FOCUS   Another well-known process is FOCUS. This model (Box 10–5) was developed by the Hospital Corporation of America (HCA), which later became known as Columbia Health Care. Once a team has focused on a single improvement opportunity, the team can then begin use of the PDCA model (JCAHO, 1992).

Joint Commission Model   The Joint Commission (JC) provides a framework for performance improvement that is both client focused and organization focused (Box 10-6). According to the JCAHO (1994), there are three components of the framework: external environment, internal environment, and cycle for improving performance. The external environment refers to the factors outside of organizations that affect the way their services are designed and implemented such as regulators, payers, and accrediting bodies. The internal environment includes the functions within organizations that affect the quality of care delivered to customers and

---

BOX 10-5 FOCUS

Find a process to improve.

Organize a team that knows the process.

Clarify current knowledge of the process.

Understand causes of process variation.

Select the process movement.

**BOX 10-6 JOINT COMMISSION CYCLE FOR
PERFORMANCE IMPROVEMENT**

Design
- Systematically determine the process's effect on the organization's mission and vision, customer expectations, and resource availability.
- Base decisions and activities on valid, reliable data.
- Involve the right people.
- Get a variety of information on the subject.

Measure
- Provide baseline data about how a process is performing.
- Gather more detailed data about how a process is functioning.
- Demonstrate the effect of an improvement action.
- Develop an organization specific performance database.

Assess
- Where can we improve?
- What are the priorities among these improvement opportunities?
- How can we improve?
- Did we improve?

Improve
- Create.
- Test.
- Implement specific innovations. (Anderson, Cuellar, & Rich, 2003.)

---

customers' perceptions of their care. The internal environment includes organization systems, management of human resources, management of information, and continuous improvement of performance. The cycle for improving performance is the main blueprint for performance improvement of functions and processes within organizations. Work on improvement can begin at any point along the cycle (JCAHO, 1995).

Six Sigma   A new entry into the health care quality industry is Six Sigma. Six Sigma, which represents three standard deviations from the mean on each end of the normal curve, is a disciplined, data-driven approach and method for eliminating "defects" or deviations. Six Sigma, as a measurement standard in product variation, can be traced back to the 1920s, when Walter Shewhart showed that three sigma (three standard deviations) from the mean is the point where a process requires correction. Many measurement standards later came on the scene, but credit for coining the term "Six Sigma" goes to a Motorola engineer named Bill Smith. The term itself is derived from statistics, whereby one tracks defects per million opportunities. A "defect" is described as anything outside of customer expectations (Chassin, 1998).

By definition, Six Sigma is less than 3.4 defects per million, or a success rate of 99.9997 percent. Given that most companies perform at a two to three sigma level (roughly 70 to 93 percent),

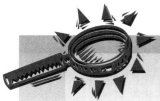

Evidence-Based Practice Box 10-1

Performance Improvement Principles Improve Orientation Program
The Franciscan Health System in Tacoma, Washington used the performance improvement model Plan-Do-Study-Act to transform their new employee orientation program from one that was not successful to one that meets their goals and is considered responsible for a decrease in employee turnover.

The project began with a needs assessment and progressed to establishment of a performance improvement team. The team agreed on objectives for success (*plan*), made changes (*do*), distributed questionnaires to new employees and considered the responses (*study*), and instituted the redesign (*act*).

Using this quality improvement model, the system has seen a significant decrease in employee turnover and an increase in employee satisfaction, suggesting that the principles of performance improvement may be adapted to a variety of health care arenas.

(Ragsdale & Mueller, 2005.)

a four sigma level, or a 99.38 percent success rate, sounds excellent. It would mean a solid "A" in school, but it would also mean that 6,210 of every million airline flights would end in disaster (Chassin, 1998).

In health care, one study revealed that only 21 percent of eligible elderly heart attack survivors were taking beta-blockers following their illness, a treatment that has been shown to save lives. According to Chassin, this represents a defect rate of 790,000 per million, or less than one sigma. In another study, Chassin found that 58 percent of clients with clinical depression were either poorly evaluated or inadequately treated, which presented a 580,000 per million defect rate. These numbers indicate health care has quite a challenge to meet a six sigma level (Chassin, 1998).

The six sigma process begins by first gaining an important understanding of one's internal and external environments. Second, but no less important, an organization must understand the needs of customers so that customer expectations can be met. The methods and quality processes used to complete six sigma projects include a systematic method for using tools, training, and measurements to facilitate the design of products and processes that meet customer expectations which can be produced at six sigma quality levels. Many of these tools are the performance improvement tools described below (Chassin, 1998).

Performance Improvement Tools Performance improvement tools are designed to help ensure that performance improvement efforts are planned and systematic, that they are based on reliable data and accurate analysis, and that they are carried out with effective teamwork and communication. These tools are grouped according to their purpose (Box 10-7).

BOX 10-7 PERFORMANCE IMPROVEMENT TOOLS

Data Capture
- Log books or other data collection instruments.
- Incident reports can be used to collect underlying causes and circumstances—these may be databased.
- Audits of medical records.
- Interviews or focus groups.
- Opinion surveys.

Data Analysis
- Control chart
- Histogram
- Run chart
- Line graph
- Scatter diagram
- Cause and effect diagram
- Flowchart

Drill Down
- Checklist or tally sheet
- Cause and effect, fishbone, or Ishikawa diagram
- Flowchart
- Pareto chart
- Scatter diagram (JCAHO, 1992.)

Examples of these statistical tools can be seen on the following pages. These tools are useful in home care; however, in-depth explanations of these tools are beyond the scope of this chapter.

Control Charts   A control chart is a run chart with upper and lower control limits on either side of the mean. These limits are based on statistical rules.

Applications
- Use when a line graph or run chart is not able to answer whether the process is out of statistical control.
- To discover whether a process is in or out of statistical control. (Variation is due to common or special causes?)

Advantages
- Monitor changes in performance.
- Ascertain causes of variation (special versus common).
- Is more sensitive than a run chart.
- Control limits usually set at three standard deviations (or sigmas) from the mean (center line).

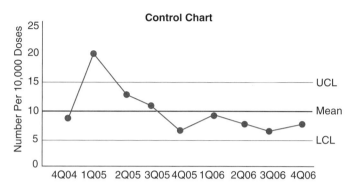

Figure 10-1 Control chart

- Different control charts are used for attribute (percentages, rates, ratios) and variable (money, time, throughput volume, scaled measurement) data.

Disadvantages
- Not easy to construct unless using statistical process control (SPC) software, and requires knowledgeable interpretation.

Figure 10-1 shows an example of a control chart.

Histograms   A histogram is a tool that shows patterns of distribution.

Applications
- Bar chart used for one variable.
- Evaluating a process at a specific moment in time.
- Used when there is a wide variety of different results.

Advantages
- Reveals whether the distribution in a process is normal, and which areas are probable causes of trouble.
- Used to visualize central location, shape, and spread of data.

Disadvantages
- Not applicable to binary (yes or no) outcomes.
- Needs a large dataset.

Figure 10-2 shows an example of a histogram.

Run Charts   A run chart plots points on a graph to show levels of performance over time.

Applications
- Used when analysis is required that is more sophisticated than a line graph, but simpler than a control chart.

Advantages
- Can indicate whether variation is due to a common or special cause.
- Quicker and easier to construct than a control chart.

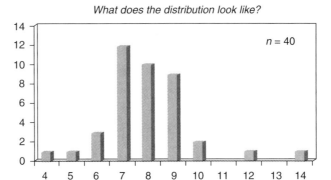

Figure 10-2 Histogram

Disadvantages

• Not as sensitive as a control chart for diagnosing outlier data.

Figures 10-3 to 10-5 show examples of run charts.

Line Graphs   A line graph is the most basic of all the performance tools. It is graphic representation of all data points.

Applications

• Used to spot trends in a process.
• Commonly used in stock market trending over time, etc.

Advantages

• Quick, easy, up-to-the-minute.

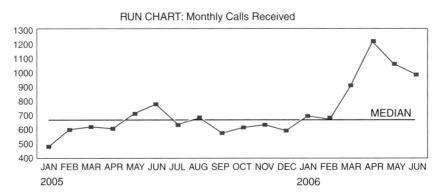

The center line in a run chart is typically the median point for the data, but some use the process average or mean as the center line

Figure 10-3 Run chart

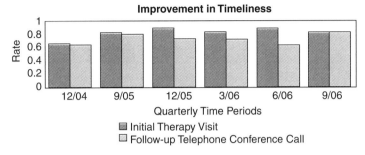

A Home Care Organization's Measures:
- Rate of initial therapy visits completed on time
- rate of f/u telephone conferences occurring on time

Figure 10-4 Run chart

Disadvantages
- Neither sophisticated nor sensitive.

Figure 10-6 gives an example of a line graph.

Scatter Diagrams A scatter diagram illustrates the relationship between variables.

Applications
- Determines whether a correlation exists between two variables—is variable A related to or affecting variable B?
- Chart searching for possible cause and effect relationship (e.g., amount of drug given, pain rating).

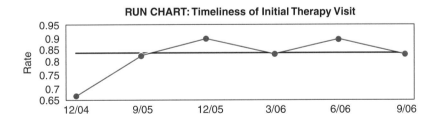

Conversion from Histogram to Run Chart

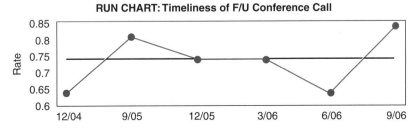

Figure 10-5 Run chart

Line Graph

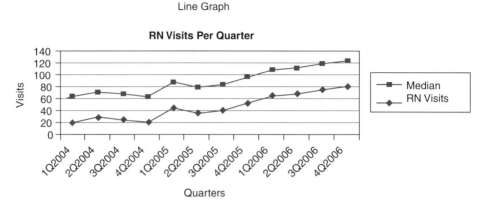

Figure 10-6 Line graph

Advantages

• Quick, easy, and certain.

Disadvantages

• Requires a large dataset.

Figures 10-7 and 10-8 give examples of scatter diagrams.

Cause and Effect, Fishbone, or Ishikawa Diagrams   A cause and effect diagram focuses on causality and shows a large number of possible causes of a particular problem or outcome.

Applications

• Early in performance improvement process.
• Assists in focusing on a number of possible causes.

Advantages

• Identify possible causes contributing to a possible problem.
• Depict the relationship between the problems and its causes.

Scatter Diagram

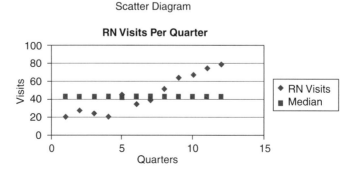

Figure 10-7 Scatter diagram

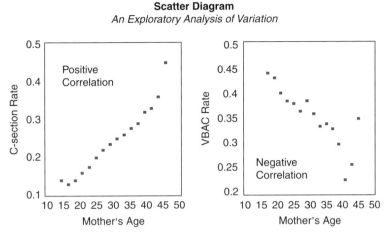

Figure 10-8 Scatter diagram

Disadvantages
- Time consuming; thought provoking, investigation needed.

Figure 10-9 shows an example of a cause and effect diagram.

Flowcharts   A flowchart depicts the sequence of steps used throughout a process.

Applications
- When designing new processes, identifying problems, planning solutions.

Advantages
- To present graphically the path a process follows, step by step.
- Helps identify inefficiencies, misunderstandings, and redundancies, while providing insight into how a given process should be performed.

Figure 10-10 shows an example of a flowchart.

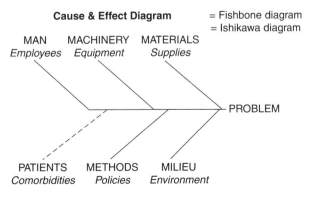

Figure 10-9 Cause and effect diagram

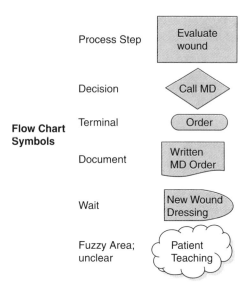

Figure 10-10 Flowchart

Outcome-Based Quality Improvement Systems

Several methods for implementing quality improvement systems in health care organizations have been developed. The Outcome Based Quality Improvement system and the Home Health Compare model were both developed by the federal government. Both methods will now be discussed.

As a part of the prospective payment system (PPS) developed for home care in 1998, the federal government implemented the Outcome Based Quality Improvement (OBQI) system (Anderson, 2000). See Chapter 7 for a discussion on PPS. The home health OBQI system consists of outcome reports generated from the Centers for Medicare and Medicaid Services (CMS), previously called the Health Care Finance Administration (HCFA), a national repository of data items specified in the Outcome and Assessment Information Set (OASIS) and reported by home health agencies to their State Survey Agencies. Under the home health OBQI System, CMS contracts with a home health support contractor that acts as a coordinating body to implement and support the system. Using OASIS outcome reports, the support contractor distributes information and guidance to all organizations participating in the system. The contractor provides education, consultation, and other technical assistance to home health agencies to help agencies develop and manage outcome-based, continuous quality improvement programs (Shaughnessy et al., 2002). For more information, please see the OASIS and Outcome-Based Quality Improvement (OBQI) in Home Health Care Report at www.cms.hhs.gov/ under the Quality Improvement section.

OBQI is a two-stage process, with the first stage being outcome analysis. For outcome analysis to be conducted for a given agency, it is necessary to collect uniform data for all clients in the agency or those clients with conditions of interest. The result of this first stage is an agency-level report showing the agency's present performance in terms of client outcomes relative to a reference sample of home care clients. This is the first outcome report, which an agency receives. The second and subsequent outcome reports contain comparisons of an agency's present performance in terms of client outcomes relative to the preceding time period for the agency and relative to a reference sample of home care clients. These outcome comparisons constitute the outcome analysis portion of OBQI. This first stage should incorporate risk adjustment through grouping or statistical methods, as appropriate. **Risk adjustment** refers to the process of compensating or controlling for the potential influence of risk factors or case mix variables that can affect outcomes (Crisler & Richard, 2002).

The outcome report produced from the first-stage analysis helps to determine which outcomes are clearly inferior and which are clearly superior relative either to the prior time period or to the reference sample. The second stage starts with those outcomes, termed target outcomes, identified for further investigation. Providers can then focus their attention and energies for quality improvement on those care behaviors that produce the target outcomes (Hausner, 2001). Reviewing care delivery for target outcomes results in findings that must be translated into recommendations for changing or reinforcing certain aspects of care provision. These recommendations are systematically documented in a plan of action for each target outcome. Once OBQI is successfully implemented in an agency and becomes a "steady-state" activity, it emerges as a powerful tool to continuously improve quality for the benefit of clients (Allen et al., 2004).

Home Health Compare

The federal government also developed Home Health Compare, a system that tracks quality measures coming from information collected by Medicare and Medicaid-certified home health agencies. The information that is collected about Medicare and Medicaid clients who get skilled care addresses the clients' health; how clients' function; the skilled care, and social, personal, and support services they need; as well as their living conditions. Home Health Compare houses the names of organizations, services provided, and benchmarking data concerning specific mandatory outcomes—outcomes that can be compared at a national and state level. The quality measures include four measures related to improvement in getting around, four measures related to meeting the client's activities of daily living, two measures related to client medical emergencies, and one measure related to improvement in mental health (Medicare, 2003a).

These quality measures are based on data collected about home health clients whose care is covered by Medicare or Medicaid and provided by a Medicare-certified home health agency. Data collected about clients serviced by a Medicaid-only certified agency, private pay clients, those under the age of 18, those receiving maternity services, and those receiving only personal care/supportive services are not submitted to the federal government. Therefore, these types of clients are excluded from the measures.

These quality measures provide information about how well home health agencies provide care for their clients. The measures provide information about clients' physical and mental health, and whether their ability to perform basic daily activities is maintained or improved. Although a client's health condition (such as heart disease or diabetes) may not be expected to improve, the client can often be expected to improve in the areas covered by the quality measures.

Quality information can be used to compare home health agencies. Hospital discharge planners, social workers, and physicians, who often help schedule the home health services, can use this information to evaluate various home health agencies. In addition to these evaluative measures, nurses can also view other home health information on this website, talk to the physician, or ask other health care professionals about their home health experiences (Medicare, 2003b.) Figure 10-11 illustrates Home Health Compare data collected for one home health agency.

Medicare Covered Services Offered						
Home Health Agency Telephone Number <u>Type of Ownership</u>	Nursing Care Services (selected)	Physical Therapy Services (selected)	Occupational Therapy Services (selected)	Speech Pathology Services (selected)	Medical Social Services (selected)	Home Health Aide Services (selected)
☑ ABCD Agency Any State, USA	✔	✔	✔	✔	✔	✔

Figure 10-11 Home Health Compare exhibit

Page Last Updated: November 25, 2003
Data Last Updated: June 21, 2004

Home Health Results

Home Health Agencies You Selected in Any State, USA

Contact Information:

1-800-Medicare	1-800-633-4227
Home Health Hotline at State Survey Agency	1-800-000-0000
State Quality Improvement Organization	1-800-000-0000

The chart(s) below gives helpful information on the agencies that you have selected. There are a total of 1 chart(s). Scroll down the page to view all of the charts for the agencies you have selected.

Be aware that: The list of home health agencies is based on the places where they have provided services in the past. Contact the home health agency to find out if they still provide services in your area.

This information (data) is gathered from the Quality Information Evaluation System (QIES). See Data Collection Details for more information.

ABCD Agency

Type of Ownership: Proprietary
Agency's Initial Date of Medicare Certification:

Medicare-covered Services:

Nursing Care Services: Yes   Speech Pathology Services: Yes
Physical Therapy Services: Yes   Medical Social Services: Yes
Occupational Therapy Services: Yes   Home Health Aide Services: Yes

Quality Measures	Percentage for ABCD HHA	State Average	National Average
HIGHER PERCENTAGES ARE BETTER			
Percentage of clients who get better at walking or moving around	38%	36%	36%
Percentage of clients who get better at getting in and out of bed	65%	49%	50%
Percentage of clients who get better at getting to and from the toilet	70%	62%	62%
Percentage of clients who have less pain when moving around	61%	56%	59%
Percentage of clients who get better at bathing	62%	58%	59%
Percentage of clients who get better at taking their medicines correctly (by mouth)	43%	40%	37%
Percentage of clients who get better at getting dressed	71%	63%	64%
Percentage of clients who stay the same (don't get worse) at bathing	91%	91%	92%
Percentage of clients who are confused less often	50%	41%	42%
LOWER PERCENTAGES ARE BETTER			
Percentage of clients who had to be admitted to the hospital	31%	35%	28%
Percentage of clients who need urgent, unplanned medical care	16%	21%	21%

Home Health Compare

Quality Measure Information

Home Health Agencies You Selected in Any State, USA

Contact Information:

1-800-Medicare   1-800-633-4227

Home Health Hotline
at State Survey Agency   1-800-000-0000

State Quality Improvement
Organization   1-800-000-0000

The following bar graphs provide helpful information for all the home health agencies that you have selected. The displays include National and State averages for each Quality Measure.

Percentage of clients who get better at walking or moving around
Why is this important?

Most people value being able to take care of themselves. In some cases, it may take more time for you to walk and move around yourself than to have someone do things for you. But, it is important that home health care staff and informal caregivers encourage you to do as much as you can for yourself. Your home health staff will evaluate your need for, and teach you how to use any special devices or equipment that you may need to help you increase you ability to perform some activities without the assistance of another person.

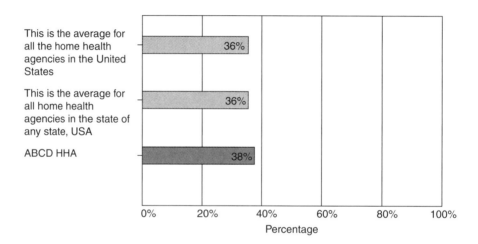

This information comes from the Home Health Outcome and Assessment Information Set (OASIS) during the time period March 2003–February 2004.

Note: The information in Home Health Compare should be looked at carefully. Use it with the other information you gather about home health agencies as you decide where to get home health services. You may want to contact your doctor, your State Survey Agency or your State Quality Improvement Organization for more information. To report quality problems, contact the State Quality Improvement Organization or State Home Health Hotline number that can be found in the **Helpful Contacts** section of this website.

Percentage of clients who get better at getting in and out of bed
Why is this important?

Most people value being able to take care of themselves. It is important that home health care staff and informal caregivers encourage you to do as much as you can for yourself. If you can get in and out of bed with little help, you may be more independent, feel better about yourself, and stay more active. This can affect your health in a good way. Your home health staff will evaluate your need for, and teach you how to use any special devices or equipment that you may need to help you increase you ability to perform some activities without the assistance of another person. Your ability to get in and out of bed yourself may help you live independently as long as possible in your own home.

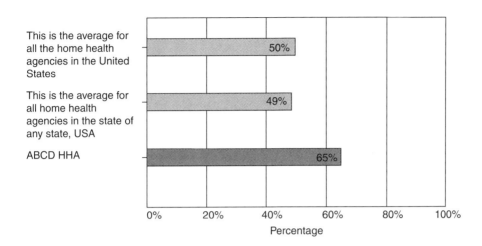

This information comes from the Home Health Outcome and Assessment Information Set (OASIS) during the time period March 2003-February 2004.

Percentage of clients who get better at getting to and from the toilet
Why is this important?

Most people value being able to take care of themselves. It may take more time for you to get to the toilet by yourself. But, it is important that home health care staff and informal caregivers encourage you to do as much as you can for yourself. Your home health staff will evaluate your need for, and teach you how to use any special devices or equipment that you may need to help you increase you ability to perform some activities without the assistance of another person.

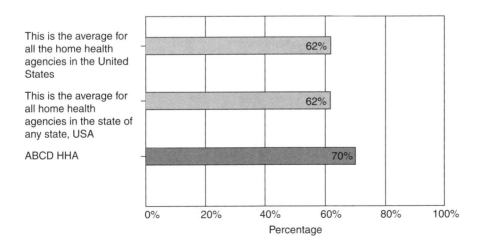

This information comes from the Home Health Outcome and Assessment Information Set (OASIS) during the time period March 2003-February 2004.

Percentage of clients who have less pain when moving around
Why is this important?

Home health staff should ask if you are having pain at each visit. If you are in pain, you (or someone on your behalf) should tell the staff. Efforts can then be made to find and treat the cause and make you more comfortable. If pain is not treated, you may not be able to perform daily routines, may become depressed, or have an overall poor quality of life. Pain may also be a sign of a new or worsening health problem.

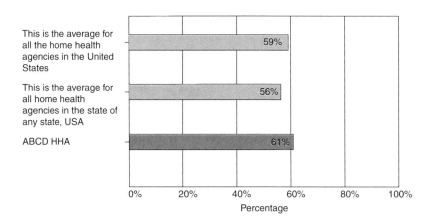

This information comes from the Home Health Outcome and Assessment Information Set (OASIS) during the time period March 2003–February 2004.

Percentage of clients who get better at bathing Why is this important?

Most people value being able to take care of themselves. In some cases, it may take more time for you to bathe yourself than to have someone bathe you. But, it is important that home health care staff and informal caregivers encourage you to do as much as you can for yourself. Your home health staff will evaluate your need for, and teach you how to use any special devices or equipment that you may need to help you increase you ability to perform some activities without the assistance of another person.

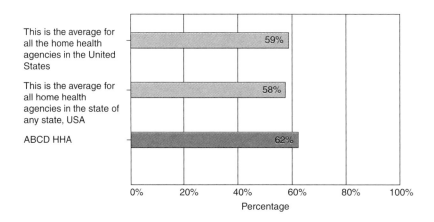

This information comes from the Home Health Outcome and Assessment Information Set (OASIS) during the time period March 2003–February 2004.

Percentage of clients who get better at taking their medicines correctly (by mouth) Why is this important?

For medicines to work properly, they need to be taken correctly. Taking too much or too little medicine can keep it from helping you feel better and, in some cases, can make you sicker, make you confused (which could affect your safety), or even cause death. Home health staff can help teach you ways to organize your medicines and take them properly. Getting better at taking your medicines correctly means the home health agency is doing a good job teaching you how to take your medicines.

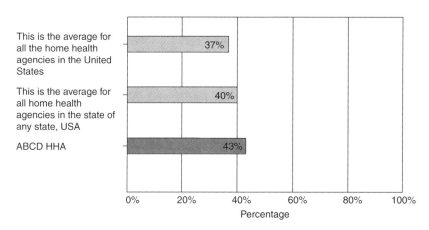

This information comes from the Home Health Outcome and Assessment Information Set (OASIS) during the time period March 2003–February 2004.

Percentage of clients who get better at getting dressed Why is this important?

Most people value being able to take care of themselves. In some cases, it may take more time for you to dress yourself than to have someone dress you. But it is important that home health staff and informal caregivers encourage you to do as much as you can for yourself. Your home health staff will evaluate your need for, and teach you how to use any special devices or equipment that you may need to help you increase you ability to perform some activities without the assistance of another person.

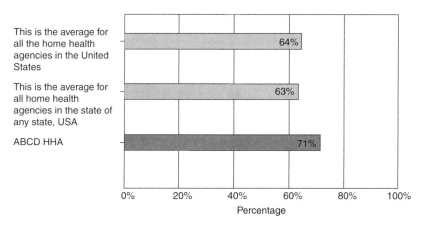

This information comes from the Home Health Outcome and Assessment Information Set (OASIS) during the time period March 2003–February 2004.

Percentage of clients who stay the same (don't get worse) at bathing
Why is this important?

Most people value being able to take care of themselves. In some cases, it may take more time for you to bathe yourself than to have someone bathe you. But, it is important that home health care staff and informal caregivers encourage you to do as much as you can for yourself. Your home health staff will evaluate your need for, and teach you how to use any special devices or equipment that you may need to help you increase you ability to perform some activities without the assistance of another person.

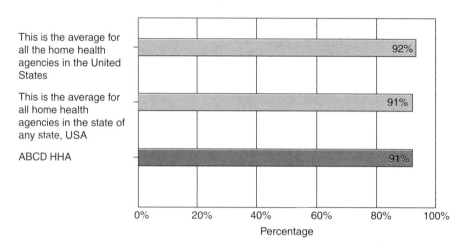

This information comes from the Home Health Outcome and Assessment Information Set (OASIS) during the time period March 2003–February 2004.

Percentage of clients who had to be admitted to the hospital Why is this important?

Some inclient hospital care may be avoided if the home health staff is doing a good job at checking your health condition at each visit to detect problems early. They also need to check how well you are eating, drinking, and taking your medicines, and how safe your home is. Home health staff must coordinate your care. This involves communicating regularly with you, your informal caregivers, your doctor, and anyone else who provides care for you.

Lower percentages are better

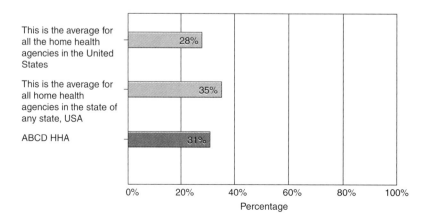

This information comes from the Home Health Outcome and Assessment Information Set (OASIS) during the time period March 2003–February 2004.

Percentage of clients who need urgent, unplanned medical care
Why is this important?

A home health care provider may refer a client to emergency care when this is the best way to treat the client's current condition. However, some emergency care may be avoided if the home health staff is doing a good job at checking your health condition to detect problems early. They also need to check how well you are eating, drinking, and taking your medicines, and how safe your home is. Home health staff must coordinate your care. This involves communicating regularly with you, your informal caregivers, your doctor, and anyone else who provides care for you.

Lower percentages are better

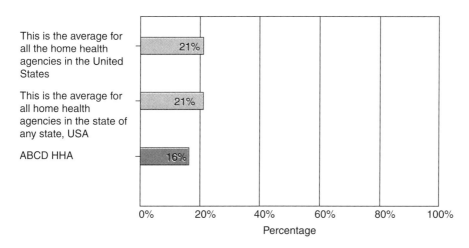

This information comes from the Home Health Outcome and Assessment Information Set (OASIS) during the time period March 2003–February 2004.

Percentage of clients who are confused less often Why is this important?

Home health staff will check you at each visit for signs of confusion. Confusion could mean you are having a reaction to a medicine or further medical problems. If you are confused, your safety may be at risk since there is more of a chance that you will take your medicines incorrectly or fall. It is important to find the cause early and treat it in the right way. If you do get confused, staff should teach you and your informal caregivers how to deal with confusion to limit its effect on the quality of your life. Usually, if you are less confused, you are better able to help take care of yourself. It is also easier for home health staff and informal caregivers to provide care to you if you are less confused.

This information comes from the Home Health Outcome and Assessment Information Set (OASIS) during the time period March 2003–February 2004.

Page Last Updated: November 03, 2003
Data Last Updated: June 21, 2004

http://www.medicare.gov/HHCompare/Search/results.asp

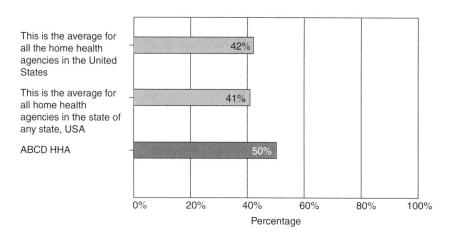

Summary

Nurses engaged in the quality/performance improvement process have found that the process is very similar to the nursing process. There are as many definitions of quality as there are health care organizations. The question that payers, clients, physicians, and health care workers must answer is twofold: what is quality and how does the organization demonstrate that quality? As has been discussed in this chapter, not only must quality definitions be selected, but those definitions must be measured, sustained, and improved through statistical processes. The processes have in common the areas of assessment, measurement, planning, and implementation.

References

Allen, B. L., Burt, P., Rochoudbury, C., & Chen, B. (2004). Analysis of OBQI outcomes in participating Michigan home health agencies. *Journal of Nursing Care Quality, 19*(2), 149-155.

Anderson, P. (2000). Thrive, survive, or perish: The impact of a prospective payment system on home health. *Policy, Politics & Nursing Practice, 2*(4), 278-283.

Anderson, P. L., Cuellar, N., & Rich, K. (2003). Performance improvement in higher education: Adapting a model from health care agencies. *Journal of Nursing Education, 42*(9), 416-420.

Barnum, B. S., & Kerfoot, K. M. (1995). *The nurse as executive.* (4th ed.). Gaithersburg, MD: Aspen.

Capezio, P. J., & Morehouse, D. L. (1993). *Taking the mystery out of TQM: A practical guide to total quality management.* Franklin Lakes, N. J.: Career Press.

Center for Medicare and Medicaid Services. (2003). OASIS and OBQI. Retrieved July 18, 2004, from http://www.cms.hhs.gov/quality/hhqi/OASIS OBQI

Chassin, M. R. (1998). Is health care ready for six sigma quality? *The Milbank Quarterly, 76*(4), 565-591.

Cosby, P. B. (1995). *Quality is still free: Making quality certain in uncertain times.* New York: McGraw-Hill.

Cosby, P. B. (1984). *Quality without tears: The art of hassle free management.* New York: Plume.

Cosby, P. B. (1979). *Quality is still free: The art of making quality certain.* New York: McGraw-Hill.

Crisler, K. S., & Richard, A. A. (2002). The basics. *Home Healthcare Nurse, 20*(8), 519-523.

Deming, W. E. (1986). *Out of crisis.* Cambridge, MA: Center for Advanced Engineering Study.

Donabedian, A. (1988). The quality of care: How can it be assessed? *Journal of the American Medical Association, 260,* 1743-1748.

Friedman, M. M. (2000). Designing home care processes to make organizational improvement: The Joint Commission Standards. *Home Healthcare Nurse, 18*(5), 292-295.

Hausner, T. (2001, February). HCFA quality improvement initiatives. *Caring Magazine,* pp. 42-43.

Joint Commission on the Accreditation of Healthcare Organizations. (1999). *Using performance measurement to improve outcomes in home care and hospice settings.* Oakbrook Terrace: Author.

Joint Commission on the Accreditation of Healthcare Organizations. (1996). *Using performance improvement tools in home care and hospice organizations.* Oakbrook Terrace: Author.

Joint Commission on the Accreditation of Healthcare Organizations. (1995). *Framework for improving performance: A guide for home care and hospice organizations.* Oakbrook Terrace: Author.

Joint Commission on the Accreditation of Healthcare Organizations. (1994). *Forms, charts, & other tools for performance improvement.* Oakbrook Terrace: Author.

Joint Commission on the Accreditation of Healthcare Organizations. (1993). *Quality improvement in home care.* Oakbrook Terrace: Author.

Joint Commission on the Accreditation of Healthcare Organizations. (1992). *Using quality assurance tools in a health care setting.* Oakbrook Terrace: Author.

Juran, J. M. (1989). *Juran on leadership for quality.* New York: Free Press.

McNeil, B. J. (2001). Stattuck lecture-hidden barriers to improvement in the quality of care. *New England Journal of Medicine, 345*(22), 1612-1620.

Medicare. (2003a). Home Health Compare. Retrieved July 18, 2004, from
http://medicare.gov/HHCompare/Home.asp?version=default browser

Medicare. (2003b). What is home health care? Retrieved July 18, 2004, from
http://www.medicare.gov/HHCompare/Home.asp?dest=NAV|Home|About#TabTop

Ragsdale, M. A., & Mueller, J. (2005). Plan, do, study, act model to improve an orientation program. *Journal of Nursing Care Quality, 20*(3), 268-272.

Richardson, W. C., & Corrigan, J. M. (2002). The IOM quality initiative: A progress report at six years. *Sharing the Future, 1*(1), 1-8.

Shaughnessy, P. W., Crisler, K. S., Hittle, D. F., & Schlenker, R. E. (2002). Summary of the report on OASIS and outcomes-based quality improvement in home care: Research and demonstration findings, policy implications, and considerations for change. *Center for Health Services Research,* March 2002, 1-6.

Walton, M. (1996). *The Deming management method.* New York: Putnam.

Chapter 11

Management of Human Resources

Ralph R. Simone, Jr.

Key Terms

Human Resources   Preceptor   Regular Staff

Per-visit Staff

A ll health care organizations are dependent upon the knowledge, intelligence, and expertise of the individuals employed in their organizations. Collectively these individuals are called the **human resources** of the organization (Huber, 2006). In the home care industry, one of the most challenging operational and client care areas is the management of human resources. The major function of human resources management in home care is the provision of qualified staff necessary for the organization to meet its clients' needs. Not only must there be a sufficient number of staff, the staff must also be competent and capable of providing the skills necessary to care for the client. Applicable skills must be updated and tested on a regular basis. This chapter will deal with providing competent staff, keeping staff competent, and retaining staff.

Recruitment of Staff

Recruitment of staff starts with knowing and understanding exactly how many staff an organization needs. To predict this number, each organization collects data in preparation for the development of a staffing plan. Organization data collected is culled from the number of client visits, number of staff, productivity, and travel factors. Staffing plans should help organizations maintain enough personnel to meet current and future demands for services. Working in conjunction with its projected business growth, an organization can then factor in the appropriate number of staff positions required to also provide care during staff illness, vacation, and other time off.

Home care agencies may work with several classifications (types) of clinical and office staff.

- **Regular staff** is made up of organizational employees who are either salaried or paid by the hour and consists of two groups:
  - Office staff, sometimes called administrative and clerical staff, are those who provide support services to the visiting staff.
  - Visiting staff, sometimes called field staff, are those who actually make home visits.
- **Per-visit staff,** who may be organizational employees or contract employees, are paid by the visit.

All the above types of staff may include registered nurses (RNs); licensed practical nurses (LPNs); certified home care aides (HHA); therapists, including physical therapists (PTs), occupational therapists (OTs), speech therapists (SPs), certified occupational therapy assistants (COTAs), and physical therapy assistants (PTAs); social workers (MSWs); pharmacists (RPHs); and others.

A correct balance of per-visit staff and regular hourly staff needs to be considered so that efficiency and the cost of care can be controlled. Through years of practice, the formula usually used to determine the staffing blend is a split of 80 percent regular staff and 20 percent per-visit staff. This split will allow an organization to ensure constant work for their regular staff while having enough flexibility with the per-visit staff to cover the visit and client fluctuations that occur in the home care business. At all times, an organization should have enough staff to fulfill its mission. As the United States moves further and further into the nursing shortage, flexibility of scheduling becomes an increasingly important tool in the recruitment of registered nurses (White, 2003).

Hiring of competent staff requires attention to many state and federal requirements. Besides legal requirements such as state licensure and I-9 documentation (to determine immigration status) other items included are:

1. Professional (not personal) references. It is extremely important to obtain, at a minimum, two professional references from an applicant's previous managers or supervisors. The organization should use a standardized form when checking references either verbally or in writing. Managers should be leery of potential employees who have difficulty supplying appropriate and recent references.
2. Physical examination. All clinical staff, regular, per-visit, and visiting, must have a pre-employment physical examination. Having the applicant aware of the physical examination requirement necessary for all clinical staff can benefit both the staff and the organization. Many times a potential employee will provide a written statement of his or her physical condition from a personal physician who may not have a full understanding of the job duties of a home care employee.

3. Criminal offender check. The criminal offender check is one of the most important pieces in the hiring process. All states have specific guidelines and rules related to restrictions of employment in health care organizations. These restrictions, based on certain types of criminal convictions, help ensure the safety of clients (as well as co-workers), and their importance cannot be overestimated.

An extensive interview with the applicant is always conducted with both a human resources (HR) representative and the potential manager within the line organization. Managers should use good judgment when hiring clinical staff. There has been an expectation that has somehow developed over time that, in home care, it is more beneficial to hire staff with acute care experience (ICU, ER) into home care positions than it is to hire inexperienced staff. There is now some debate as to whether it might not be just as acceptable to hire the more inexperienced nurse and mentor him or her in the area of home care. Home care, as has been previously discussed in other chapters, is an altogether different type of clinical care than acute care, and previous experience may not always be an asset.

Although home care certainly offers more flexibility than acute care, it is not easier. A home care nurse needs to be able to function independently and at all times have excellent judgment skills. An initial review of credentials and qualifications is a must prior to hiring an applicant for employment in home care. One of the most important qualifications to be examined prior to hiring is state licensure and exclusions from the Medicare program. When individuals have been found guilty of Medicare fraud, they may be excluded from providing any services to Medicare patients; as a result, any agency that uses their service would not be reimbursed. This can be a problem for agencies that provide services to Medicare recipients.

Orientation, Training, and Education

A detailed and extensive orientation is the first step in the continuous training and education of a professional staff member. Orientation generally covers three areas:

- An overview of the organization, its mission, and its services.
- The general organization policies and procedures, such as the Health Insurance Portability and Accountability Act (HIPAA) and client rights. Many state, federal, and JC-specific policies would be included in the orientation program.
- A focus on the competencies and clinical skills needed to work within the home care environment. These competencies are determined by the agency based on the services provided. An example would be an agency that provides skilled nursing care of patients receiving chemotherapy. That agency would do specific competencies concerning biohazard management differently than an agency that does not provide those services.

Organization Mission Statement

An organization's mission statement usually identifies the organization's reason for being. Generally, in home care, the mission statement will make reference to quality care, client and family education and involvement in decision making, maintenance of current health status, and helping clients and families cope with issues of health care and possibly death. A sample mission statement appears in Box 11-1.

BOX 11-1 Long Beach Home Care Mission Statement

The mission of Long Beach Home Care is to, in a caring and compassionate manner, provide clients and their families quality health care services, educate clients and their families about health care options, involve clients and their families in their care, and prepare clients and their families for self-care, discharge, and possibly a peaceful death.

General Organization Policies

The organization policy section should focus on such items as the Abuse and Neglect Policy; the Confidentiality Policy, inclusive of (HIPPA) regulations; and Client Rights and Responsibilities. New employees also need to understand standard precautions such as those for blood-borne pathogens, TB precautions, and infection-control reporting. Review of organization policies on safety, security, corporate compliance, problem resolution, and emergency preparedness are also included in the policy review. A signed acknowledgment sheet stating that the new employee received training and materials on all facets covered during orientation is essential. An important feature of this section would be the dissemination and review of an Employee Handbook if one is used.

Competencies

The last piece of orientation deals with clinical competencies. This critical piece ties in with the continuing education of professional staff. Each year, the clinical organization reviews clinical data related to service utilization, adverse events, performance improvement, and federal and state compliance issues that had the most occurrences during the previous year. From this data, clinical competency instruction and testing is developed.

There are always four areas of competency testing that are mandatory for all clinical staff. Those areas include infection control, national client safety standards, client rights and confidentiality, and advance directives. The same competencies are also taught and tested during orientation for new staff, so that all staff is "on the same page" (Joint Commission on Accreditation of Heathcare Organizations, 2006).

In addition to the competency testing just described, all clinical staff should complete a set of skill tests specific to their discipline. For nurses, these skills commonly include client assessment, specific types of wound care, infusion skills, and many other skills. Also, if during the course of employment, a new skill is required to be performed by the clinical staff, the need for additional education and competency testing could result in a midyear competency evaluation. Accurate and complete records of completed competencies are kept in the employee's personnel file and may be reviewed by federal and state agencies and by accrediting bodies.

Preceptorship

Preceptor programs have proven to be a factor in increasing retention rates in health care organizations (Baggot, Hensinger, & Parry, 2005). After the initial orientation, some agencies place new employees with a **preceptor**. A preceptor is a professional employed in a practice setting who is assigned to work alongside a student or new employee for purposes of teaching/learning (Mamchur & Myrick, 2003). It is not uncommon for a new employee to spend four to six weeks working closely with an assigned preceptor. Preceptors are generally top clinical employees who not only have excellent clinical skills but also excellent teaching and communication skills. Preceptors are chosen very carefully. Being chosen as a preceptor should be viewed by the staff as a validation of excellence in clinical practice. Some organizations provide additional compensation for being named a preceptor. This is a way for senior management to demonstrate their commitment to excellence in clinical practice. Whether or not an increase (or differential) is given, clinicians should be proud of their preceptor status (Lawless, Demers, & Baker, 2002).

Finally, training is not just an orientation event. In-services are provided throughout the year to keep staff updated on specific work-related issues and to increase staff knowledge. Every year, the staff development division of the organization should use various data from the previous year to determine which competencies need to be covered. Merging data from incidents that have occurred, new developments in specific areas, and discussions with the clinical management team determine the types of new or additional services that may be provided the next year. By focusing on current and pertinent issues, well-selected in-services can prepare clinicians and organizations to be equipped to confront difficult issues that they may face in the future.

Retention of Staff

The most effective way of providing adequate staffing within an organization is for the organization to keep the staff that it has. Keeping turnover at a minimum not only provides adequate staffing to the organization, it keeps morale high, and can help control operating costs. The less hiring done, the more cost effective an organization will be. Less hiring also means less advertising, less training, and a better trained and more experienced staff. The money saved from turnover can be used to provide raises for the clinical staff or to purchase new equipment such as computers to make their jobs more efficient.

The national average for registered nurse (RN) turnover in home care is 18.82 percent, and for licensed practical nurses (LPNs) is over 22 percent (Hospital & Health Care Compensation Services, 2003–2004). For an organization with 150 RNs, this means that over a year's time, 28 employees would have to be replaced. For larger organizations, the impact is even greater. This is not only costly but extremely time consuming.

Several reasons have been sited as variables in nurse turnover and in nurses' intentions to leave their nursing positions. Most, in one way or another, are correlated to job satisfaction. Job commitment, adequate staffing, and job setting have been shown to have a positive influence in reduction in turnover (Shaver, & Lacey, 2003). Additionally, the influence of mentoring, staff development, and the manager's role have also been cited as contributors to job satisfaction. However, in comparing job employment arenas, home health nurses were among those most satisfied (Rambur et al., 2003).

The first step in staff retention is finding out why employees are leaving. Of course, this does not include involuntary terminations or what is generally acknowledged as "good turnover." One key to this data collection is the exit interview. Most exiting employees will divulge exactly why they are leaving. Less verbal exiting employees may offer useful information if interviewed properly. This data needs to be collected and analyzed so that appropriate organizational changes can be made. Some administrators suggest that, rather than

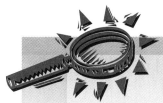

Evidence-Based Practice Box 11-1

Adoption of Magnet Programs in Home Care May Help with Recruitment and Retention of Nurses

The nursing shortage in the United States is expected to continue, making recruitment and retention of nurses an ongoing concern. Insufficient enrollment in nursing schools and the aging RN workforce are but two contributors to the problem. The problem is especially urgent in home care, where the nursing workforce will need to double by 2020.

(Flynn, 2003)

Research related to the Magnet Recognition Hospital Program sponsored by the American Nurses Credentialing Center suggests that the program, which fosters excellence in nursing services through a professional nursing atmosphere, is a positive factor in both the recruitment and retention of registered nurses. It has further been suggested that home care organizations, nurses, and consumers could all benefit from magnet recognition. The time is right for home care agencies to implement a program whose success is well documented in research and practice.

(Brady-Schwartz, 2005; Flynn, 2003; Frazier, 2003)

ask staff why they are leaving, an effective retention strategy is to ask staff why they stay (Hill & Ingala, 2002).

Exit Interview

Consistency can be gained by creating an exit interview questionnaire so that the same and most pertinent questions will be asked by whoever is conducting the exit interview. A third party (not the manager from the exited department) should conduct the exit interview, so that data will be shared freely. In most cases, human resources professionals conduct the exit interviews.

As an example of reacting positively to a retention problem, one organization collected data that showed that about 40 percent of its turnover took place within the first year of employment. There was no significant data that indicated why this was happening. To help the organization create a process that would reduce the turnover, a tool was developed to determine why this was happening. Understanding why was the first step in the solution.

The organization developed a tool that would allow pertinent data to be collected. It then developed a process in which all new employees met with and were interviewed by an HR representative (generally speaking, the person that hired them) after the first month of employment. This quickly proved to be much too soon after hire to gather meaningful data. Employees were still in training and learning the basics of the job, so it was too soon for them to provide administration with meaningful data. The timeframe was changed to two months after hiring, which would allow the new employee to have a better feel of the organization and the work being done. Specifically, data were gathered on the following subjects:

- Orientation process
- Tools
- Manager/supervisor
- Preceptor process
- Scheduling process
- Recognition/retention
- Surprises
- Concerns
- The organization in general

By using this data, the organization was able to change some of its processes and provide more support for the new clinical staff. As a result, one-year turnover decreased. (Homecare Foundation, 2005).

It is extremely important that data gathered be used to solve problems and not to point fingers at individuals. If a new hire is having trouble with her or his supervisor, that information needs to be shared in a way that will help the supervisor learn, and not threaten the employee who passed on the information. Information gathered this way must only be used to coach and improve, not discipline. Although individual information of any importance must be shared immediately, the complete data should be reviewed at the senior management level periodically, with specific plans made to solve major reoccurring issues. The new data can be combined with data compiled from exit interviews to garner a total picture of turnover for the organization. As a result, the organization in the example above has a turnover rate in the RN field of an incredibly low 6 percent. In fact, turnover for the entire population of this organization is less than 16 percent. This saves money (hiring, orienting, preceptoring, advertising) while continuing to provide consistent, quality client care.

Employment Satisfaction Survey

Another tool used to help retain staff is an annual employee satisfaction survey. Our target organization developed its survey tool in 1999, and it has been used annually since that date. The tool continues to use the same 30 questions each year. The questions cover all aspects of work life at the organization. It is important to generally keep the same questions so that trend progress or declination of scores can be monitored through the years. The questions focus on the major items that an organization may want to measure, such as morale, training, compensation, and benefits. Selecting five or six major categories, and developing five or six questions about each result, assists in obtaining the desired information. Keeping the survey simple also helps in getting employees to complete it. Using a simple Likert scale of "agree, disagree, and neutral" helps to provide discrete data yet the data is not so discrete as to require too much analysis (Homecare Foundation, 2005; SPSS Techniques Series, 2006).

The process should be uncomplicated and followed each year to ensure consistency (JCAHO, 2006). At the same time each year, the organization's leader sends all employees a letter with the survey attached. The letter requests that each and every employee take the time to complete the survey. Of course, the survey is confidential, and therefore does not include the employee's name or signature. A variety of methods may be used to collect and sort the data. Data is usually segregated by:

1. Department
2. Professional visiting staff
3. Paraprofessional staff
4. Administrative staff
5. Management/supervisory
6. Length of service

This method allows administrators to review the data and pinpoint areas of concerns, both within an individual department or job category, as well as globally throughout the organization. Starting each spring, the process becomes a circular one that includes the following steps:

1. Survey mailed, returned, and data compiled.
2. Survey results presented to senior management.
3. Items of concern from previous year reviewed.
4. Areas of concern identified from current survey results.
5. Appropriate focus groups formed to address specific issues identified with the information made available to all employees via memo, presentations, "road shows," and team meetings.
6. Changes, made as a result of the focus groups, are communicated to all employees.
7. Each spring, the process is started again at step 1.

Probably the most important facet of the "survey circle" is using employees as parts of solutions. As a result of this process the organization is better able to focus its resources on significant opportunities for improvement. This is important so that employees do not feel that they are being patronized with a "morale survey" that never results in issues or problems being resolved. A promise should never be made that can't be kept! There is no quicker way to ensure nonparticipation in a survey than by not correcting issues and not communicating back to employees. Remember, this process is a circle.

Management Visibility

Finally, administrators should be seen by their staff, should be encouraged to ask questions, and should seek answers to staff questions. There is nothing worse than leaving a question unanswered. Unanswered questions will leave employees feeling that administrators are afraid to answer them. Staff should be updated on what is happening within their organization. There is possibly nothing more frustrating than allowing employees' minds to wander, thereby inviting speculation and guesses about what is going on. The scenario that an employee develops mentally will not be a positive one, and it will certainly not be the correct one. If employees believe that management is not talking to them, they will believe that it is because the news is bad. Remember, it's never as bad as thought, and it is always easier to deal with truths than perceptions.

Personnel Records

One of the more mundane pieces of the human resources management process is the maintenance of personnel records. This is an area where anything less than 100 percent is not acceptable. Files need to be audited on a regular basis. A simple monthly process (number of files divided by 12) will ensure the accuracy that is required in this area. Additionally, files should be arranged in easy to access sections with all necessary information available to anyone with authorized access. A suggestion is to have the HR files sectioned off into four or five sections. The first section would include new hire paperwork (application, references, offer letter, Medicare Sanction List, Nurses Aide Registry, driver's license, and auto insurance).

The second section can include all licensure information and competency tests. A third section would have such items as Occupational Safety and Health Administration (OSHA) requirements, confidentiality statements, and receipt of the organization handbook. Evaluations and/or supervisions could be section four and section five might include inservice data and other education and training information. Criminal background checks and I-9 information are kept separate, as is health care information. All files and data must be kept locked in a secured area. Exactly how the information is organized is not as important as its being organized so that all information is easily accessible to appropriate organization members.

Summary

The management of organizations' human resources is every manager's responsibility. Without the first-line supervisor, the senior manager or executive is powerless to retain employees. If retaining employees is not a priority, then providing competent staff to meet the needs of clients will have very little chance of happening. It is an effort that must take place every day. From the very top of an organization to the entry-level supervisor, it is every manager's responsibility to coach, groom, support, educate, and retain staff. Plus, it is not just their staff, but also every staff member in every position in every piece of the organization.

Employees must have trust and respect for virtually every manager in an organization. It has been said that one of the biggest complaints of employees was management's inability to deal with poor performance. In the experience of this author-manager, it has been found that if you *tell* employees what to do, about 25 percent will do the task as requested. If you *ask* employees to perform a task, about 50 percent will perform the task appropriately. However, if employees *participate* in the resolution of a problem, almost 100 percent will perform accordingly.

These strategies will retain employees and will ultimately allow an organization to reach its mission statement. That is what the management of human resources is truly all about.

References

Baggot, D. M., Hensinger, B., & Parry, J. (2005). Then new hire/preceptor experience. *Journal of Nursing Administration, 35*(3), 138–145.

Brady-Schwartz, D. C. (2005). Further evidence on the magnet recognition program: Implications for nursing leaders. *Journal of Nursing Administration, 35*(9), 397–403.

Flynn, L. (2003). Agency characteristics most valued by home care nurses: Findings of a nationwide study. *Home Healthcare Nurse, 21*(1), 812–817.

Frazier, S. C. (2003). Magnet home care agencies: A professional way to impact quality and retention. *Home Healthcare Nurse, 21*(9), 603–610.

Hill, K., & Ingala, J. (2002). Just ask them. *Nursing Management, 33*(10), 21–22.

Homecare Foundation. (2005). Lawrence, MA.

Hospital & Health Care Compensation Services. (2003-2004). *Home care Salary and Benefits Report.*

Huber, D. (2006). *Leadership & nursing care management* (3rd ed.). Philadelphia: Saunders.

Joint Commission on the Accreditation of Healthcare Organizations. (2006). 2006-2007 Comprehensive accreditation manual of home care. Oakbrook Terrace: Author.

Lawless, R. P., Demers, K, A., & Baker, L. (2002). Preceptor program boosts recruitment & retention. *Caring, 21*(9), 10-12.

Mamchur, C., & Myrick, F. (2003). Preceptorship and interpersonal conflict: A multidisciplinary study. *Journal of Advanced Nursing, 43*(2), 188-196.

Rambur, B., Palumbo, M. V., McIntosh, B., & Mongeon, J. (2003). A statewide analysis of RN's intention to leave their position. *Nursing Outlook, 51*(4), 182-188.

Shaver, K. H., & Lacey, L. M. (2003). Job and career satisfaction among staff nurses. *Journal of Nursing Administration, 33*(3), 166-172.

SPSS Techniques Series. *Statistics on Likert Scale Surveys.* Retrieved October 18, 2006, from http://www.uni.edu/its/us/document/stats/spss2.html

White, K. (2003). Effective staffing as a guardian of care. *Nursing Management, 34*(7), 20-25.

Chapter 12

Informatics and Technology

Deolinda Mignor, RN, DNS

Key Terms

Distant Site	Informatics	Point-of-Care (POC) Documentation
Home Telehealth	Nursing Informatics	

The collection, communication, and storage of client information are crucial aspects of health care. Organizational changes within the health care industry have driven the need for nurses with enhanced electronic communication skills and an increased reliance for health care delivered in the home (Russo, 2001). Within the last decade there has been a technological wave that has revolutionized the way data is managed within the industry. In home care, the traditional medical record or chart has been replaced with computerized records; and pagers, voicemail, cell phones, personal digital assistants, and laptops are as much a part of the home care nurse's equipment as is the stethoscope (Struk, 2001).

Until recently, client exposure to health care technology has mainly taken place in traditional settings such as hospitals and outpatient clinics. Ultrasound and magnetic resonance imaging techniques are familiar to most people, but they may not think of these devices as technology. Technology in the home or elsewhere for use by home care clients presents an entirely different picture than technology in acute care settings.

Computer technology has enabled the telecommunication industry to grow so rapidly that the way health care information is now gathered, communicated, and stored has given rise to the term **home telehealth.** Home telehealth refers to remote care delivery or monitoring between a health care provider and a client outside of a clinical health facility, usually the home (Chetney, 2003b).

Traditionally, when home care clients were assessed, visited, or cared for by a home care nurse, it meant an in-person visit to the home of the client. Today, many of the same visits may be done from a **distant site** using computer technology. A distant site is defined as the place where the health care provider is located at the time the service is delivered via a telecommunication system (U.S. Department of Health and Human Services, 2003).

This chapter will discuss the history of computer technology, telehealth, and informatics in the health care industry and home care in particular; the types of telecommunication and other technology available to home care agencies; the advantages and disadvantages of each; the reaction of nurses and clients to telehealth in home care; and a look to the future.

History of Informatics in Health Care

The term **informatics**, originated in the 1970s, meant computer processing of data and information. In nursing, this process, known as **nursing informatics** has broadened to include not only processing information but also computer technology and computer systems that transform input data to output information (Saba, 2001). Nursing informatics generated widespread interest and appeal among nurses who were able to envision the possibilities of technological advances in nursing. The American Nurses Association (ANA) approved nursing informatics as a specialty in 1992 and has since developed the ANA Standards and Scope of Nursing Informatics (ANA, 2001).

The definition of nursing informatics (NI) has changed several times as the field has evolved. The earliest NI definitions, which appeared as early as 1980, emphasized the application of computer technology to nursing. New and more complex definitions have evolved due to the newness of NI as an independent specialty. The most current definition of NI from the American Nurses Association is:

> a specialty that integrates nursing science, computer science, and information science to manage and communicate data, information, and knowledge in nursing practice. Nursing informatics facilitates the integration of data, information and knowledge to support clients, nurses, and other providers in their decision-making in all roles and settings. This support is accomplished through the use of information structures, information processes, and information technology. (2001, p. 17.)

In this chapter the term nursing informatics is used in a wide sense to encompass all information generated related to the home care client.

Assessment of Client Needs

There are several types and levels of informatic devices available to home care providers. This discussion, related to client assessment, addresses information that will be obtained via telehealth. As with all other equipment used in home care either by the nurse or by the client, the first step is assessment of the client to determine if the telehealth equipment is a *good fit* for the situation.

The assessment of the home care client prior to initiating a telehealth (distant site) program includes the client's "(a) ability to use the telehealth equipment regularly and correctly, (b) level of communication skills, (c) willingness to use the equipment, and (d) ability to follow medication schedules, dietary regimes and other care plan components" (Kinsella, 2003, p. 662).

Clients' medical conditions and states of health should be included when assessing their suitability for entry into a plan of care that includes telehealth. It has been established that the care of clients with diabetes; heart disease, especially congestive heart failure; and mental health diagnoses, such as schizophrenia and post-traumatic stress disorder, have improved with the use of telehealth devices in their homes (Chetney, 2003a; Kinsella, 2003; Kobb, Hilsen, & Ryan, 2003).

Types of Informatics/Technology in Home Care

Informatics/technology in health care may be divided into those technologies that do not use computers and those technologies that require a computer. Telehealth monitoring and videophones are examples of noncomputer technologies, and immediate documentation of client care, known as **point-of-care (POC) documentation**, is an example of informatics/technology that requires a computer. Point-of-care documentation is so named because documentation is initiated and completed at the exact point (time) when the client care is delivered.

Noncomputer Technologies

Noncomputer technologies, sometimes referred to as telehealth devices, include audio monitors, audio and video monitors, in-home messaging devices, and digital cameras. None of these technologies require a phone line or a wireless connection.

Tele-Home Care   Tele-home care refers to monitoring or visiting a home care client via a phone line or a wireless connection. The equipment, referred to as monitors, may be only audio, or may be audio and video. Both versions use sensing devices to transmit data to the home care agency, which is sometimes referred to as a station. The most common assessments done via a tele-home monitor are vital signs including blood pressure, weight, lung sounds, and O_2 saturation levels (Tweed, 2003). It is noteworthy to mention that home monitoring of obstetrical clients for assessment of premature contractions and fetal heart rates has been done for years (Figure 12-1).

Telemonitors and Videophones   Telemonitors and videophones also allow off-site visiting and monitoring of home care clients. These systems, which use a telephone line or wireless connection, have the added dimension of a two-way video connection. Chetney describes the monitor as about "the size of a large bread box" (2003b, p. 682). Nurses control the two-way audiovisual connectivity by initiating the visit, which may be a short visit or a complete home visit, except that the nurse is not in the client's home. Full video capacity enables the client to see the nurse, and the nurse to see the client (Chetney, 2003b; Tweed, 2003).

Messaging Devices   A home-messaging device is a phone line instrument that helps home care clients to manage their health plan of care. The devise, which plugs into a phone with a standard phone jack, looks like and is about the size of a digital clock. Although home care nurses have long been calling their clients at home to remind them about aspects of their care, such as their medication schedules, home messaging devices do not require the nurse to

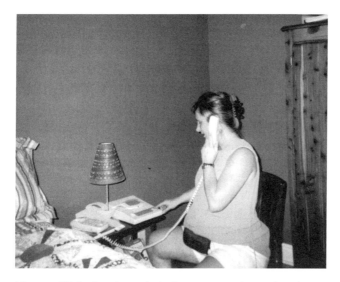

Figure 12-1 An obstetrical client uses a telemonitor for assessment of premature contractions.

call the client. There are many products available for in-home use; however, the products have similar features and the goal of all is improvement of client health outcomes.

Some home messaging devices will assess the client by having the client call a toll-free number that answers with a recording that asks specific questions related to the client's diagnosis. The client will answer the questions by using the numbers on a touch-tone phone. Other versions will call the client's home at specific times to remind the client about medications, nutrition, or other aspects of care. Home messaging devices have proven to be useful assistants for helping home care clients, especially the elderly, to be compliant in their plans of care (Kobb, Hilsen, & Ryan, 2003).

Digital Cameras   Polaroid cameras, long a part of the home care nurse's equipment, have been replaced with the digital camera. The most frequent use of the digital camera by the home care nurse is to supplement wound documentation. Although a photograph does not eliminate the need for the usual wound assessment data of location, size, and depth, it does enhance standard wound documentation.

A more recent use of the digital camera in the home relates to client safety. Goal number one of the JC 2006 Home Care National Patient Safety Goals is "Improve the accuracy of patient identification" (2005, p. 1). With this safety mandate from JC, some home care agencies have begun to include in client records a picture of the client (JCAHO, 2005; P. Anderson, personal interview, Nov. 29, 2005).

Digital cameras are within the budget range of home care agencies and have become standard equipment of the home care nurse. Most digital cameras include software that allows images to be downloaded to the nurse's laptop computer.

Point-of-Care Documentation

Regulatory and reimbursement demands have forced home care agencies to streamline the way that their client data is collected. Many agencies have acknowledged that the way to make their systems more efficient, while improving their home care delivery systems, is to initiate a point-of-care (POC) documentation system. The health care provider who uses a POC documentation system is not recording the client visit on paper, but rather is documenting the visit on a laptop computer. This information system, which can be used by all health practitioners, is replacing manual documentation.

Home care agencies started using laptops in the 1980s. Acceptance of laptops was slow, and in 2003 it was estimated that only about 25 percent of home care clinicians were carrying mobile computers (Joch, 2003), a percentage that has steadily increased since then.

Nurses and clients alike have expressed apprehension about POC documentation. Most concerns center around fears that clients perceive their importance may become secondary to the computer, a situation that is worrisome to all involved in POC documentation (Struk, 2001). However, POC anxieties diminish as nurses increase their technical skills and comfort level with their laptops. In recent years there has been a surge of interest and implementation of POC documentation.

Point-of-care documentation on a laptop, which begins with a password and ends at the agency office (station), enables home care nurses to:

- Start the day by checking their scheduled visits.
- Review recent client visits by other care team members.
- Assess the client and record all assessment data.
- Review the physician's plan of care.
- Review all medications and research on a medication database for possible medication interactions or contraindications.
- Send documentation directly to the station (agency office), thereby instantly making the information available to other team members. (Joch, 2003; Stricklin et al., 2000; Struk, 2002b).

The following scenario follows a home care nurse through her day. Susan is about to begin her day as a home care nurse for a large home care agency. She turns on her laptop by entering her password, and immediately her schedule for the day appears on the screen. Her first client is not new to her, so there is no need to seek directions to the client's home. Once in the client's home, she enters a second password that will bring her to the clinical screen and the view tree or menu. The menu allows her the option of clicking on individual screens that display the client's medications, physician orders, notes recorded from previous visits, or the client's demographics. Today, because her client has a diabetic leg ulcer, she clicks on *wound note*. The note will appear on the screen, and Susan will record the wound-related data on the note. This visit will include taking a picture of the wound with a digital camera that will be scanned into the client's electronic record.

Susan knows that this client is not comfortable with the POC documentation, so she carefully watches for signs of distress from the client that may indicate he is tiring. Susan makes a point of paying more attention to the client than to the laptop. At the completion of the POC visit, Susan locks the note, which will later (within eight hours) be transmitted to the station (agency), and she is ready for her next visit (Figures 12-2 and 12-3).

As Susan leaves the client's home, the home care aide (HCA) arrives to begin her visit. Upon entering the home, the HCA keys in her number via phone, letting the system know where she is. This process, known as telephony, allows the station to know the location of their aides, a benefit that not only is efficient for the agency's clerical staff but also serves as a safety measure for the HCA. Upon completion of the visit, the HCA notes are also entered via telephony. Because each segment of care delivered, such as bed bath, linen change, or

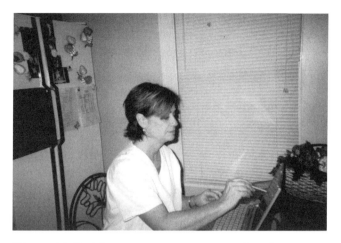

Figure 12-2 A home care nurse enters point-of-care documentation in the client's home.

shampoo, is identified by code, the HCA has only to enter the appropriate code and the HCA note is processed, eliminating the need for paper documentation.

Personal Digital Assistants

Personal digital assistants (PDAs) are small versions of laptop computers; in spite of their small size, they have many of the same functions as their larger counterparts. PDAs have become popular as the general public has begun to recognize their abilities in organizing and managing busy life-styles. In addition to personal organizing, PDA functions include voicemail, e-mail, digital photography, data and document storage, music players, and Adobe Acrobat Reader.

Home care nurses lead busy and sometimes hectic days as they travel to and from their home care clients while keeping track of scheduling, changes in client conditions, volumes of

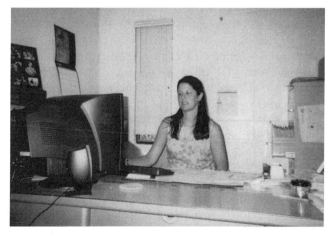

Figure 12-3 Point-of-care documentation is received at the home care agency.

data, and a great deal of other information related to the delivery of nursing care. Use of PDAs by home care nurses does not replace laptop POC documentation, but PDAs offer additional assistance to the busy home care nurse. PDA functions that may be of help to the home care nurse include the following:

- Nursing pharmaceutical reference books that include general drug guides, herbal preparation guides, and antibiotic guides.
- Guides related to diagnoses.
- Medical dictionaries and glossaries.
- Lab reference guides.
- Photography options.
- Language translation.
- Agency documents like schedules and maps. (Smith-Stoner, 2003.)

Advantages of Information Technology in Home Care

The rate of growth of information technology, which includes point-of-care documentation, telephone, and telehealth monitors in the home, is expected to increase (Chetney, 2003a; Lewis, 2001; Tweed, 2003). The effects of the technological movement in health care delivery have touched health care delivery professionals, clients, and caregivers. Nowhere are the effects more evident than in home care.

Clients

Improved client care and an increase in people taking an active role in their own health care are important advantages of computer technology and telehealth in the home. Computer technology, especially the Internet, offers all computer-literate people health-related information at their fingertips, and with the millions of soon to be retired people in the United States, the number of computer literate people over the age of 65 years will increase (Lewis, 2001). The means that more home care clients and their caregivers will be looking to technology for information support.

Many examples of improved client care and maintenance through the use of telemonitoring have been cited. Especially successful are those programs that monitor clients with chronic congestive heart failure (CHF). Telehealth programs have enabled home care nurses to identify impending CHF exacerbations by telemonitoring blood pressure and weight. Improved outcomes for diabetic clients, both in wound care and in managing glucose levels, have also been attributed to telemonitoring. The introduction of telemonitoring has been successful in reducing the number of hospitalizations and emergency room visits, reducing the number of hospital days, and increasing client satisfaction among home care clients. Additionally, there are reports that indicate clients demonstrate an improvement in their self-help attitudes and in their general feelings of well-being as a result of being part of telehealth monitoring (Chetney, 2003a; Jerant, Azari, & Nesbitt, 2001; Kinsella, 2003; Lewis, 2001; Lupoli & Rizzo, 2003).

Home care clients who live in rural communities or in large rural states benefit from nursing informatics and computer technology. Where in the past, time and distance may have

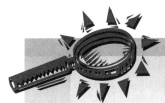

Evidence-Based Practice Box 12-1

Computer Intervention Improved Psychosocial Health

Chronic illness requires life adaptations that may cause emotional stress. This may be more troublesome for people who live in rural areas, where social contact is limited. An experimental research study by Hill and co-workers (2006) sought to determine the impact of a computer-delivered intervention on a group of 100 women with chronic illnesses living in the rural northwest. Areas addressed were social support, self-esteem, empowerment, self-efficacy, stress, depression, and loneliness, which together are considered factors that influence the success of activities that promote good mental health.

The women in the experimental group participated in a 22-week program of online peer-led support groups and online teaching units. The women also were able to communicate with each other via chat rooms and e-mail.

Study results comparing the experimental group with the control group indicated that the computer interventions were very helpful to the participants, especially in the areas of self-esteem, social support, and empowerment. Results for the other factors (depression, loneliness, and stress) suggested that over time all participants changed but did not differ statistically.

This study is of interest to home care nurses who often must limit client visits or even discharge their clients before they have come to grips with their chronic illnesses. Knowing that computer interventions have proven successful in dealing with both the negative aspects of a chronic illness and the isolation associated with rural life may encourage home care nurses to suggest this intervention to their clients.

made in-person home care visits problematic for both clients and providers, telehealth through messaging or video visits keep rural home care clients in touch with their home care providers (Dimmick et al., 2004; Kinsella, 2003; Lewis, 2001).

Caregivers

Advantages of computer technology and telehealth to caregivers include not only the possibility for greater communication with home care professionals, but also the opportunity to communicate with other caregivers. There are approximately 44.4 million caregivers in the United Stated. This represents 21 percent of the adult population in an estimated 22.9 million households. It is well known that caregivers often experience depression and a sense of burden as a result of their caregiver roles (Mignor, 2000; National Alliance for Caring & AARP, 2004). Caregivers need encouragement and affirmation that they are doing a good job. Communication with the home care professional can supply the caregiver with much-needed and appreciated emotional support. A client's positive response to telemonitoring will not only help the client but also the client's caregiver.

Home Care Professionals

The benefits of computer technology to the home care professional, although many and varied, begin with improved client care. It is computer technology that enables all caregivers—nurses, therapists, home care aides, and office personnel—who are involved in a specific client's plan of care, to be involved in the coordination of that care, in spite of different schedules. Health histories and related background information such as medication regimes and previous professional home visits by other clinicians are instantly available to the health provider, as is the current record and plan of care. Nurses can care for their clients without being in their homes, an advantage that is particularly attractive in rural states where travel time is long and costly (Stazesky, 2003).

The sharpness and accuracy of video telemonitoring, through off-site visualization of infusion sites and wounds, has eliminated unnecessary in-person visits by specialty nurses. This, in turn, allows for better efficiency and speedier responses of specialty nurses when an in-person visit is needed (Lupoli & Rizzo, 2003).

Nursing informatics and the Internet have been successful in helping home care agencies and individual nurses meet ongoing educational needs. Many health care organizations have experienced a decrease in funding for education. Where it was once possible to send professional staff to conferences, workshops, and courses, it is now necessary to find other means for staff to participate in educational programs. For some, educational programs are necessary to earn continuing education units to maintain licenses and certifications. For others, educational programs are necessary for maintaining mastery in specialty areas (Long et al., 2000).

The Internet can offer programs that meet continuing education needs. Many colleges and universities offer online courses, both for credit and not for credit, and some offer entire degree programs online. The educational possibilities resulting from the union of nursing informatics and computer technology are endless.

Disadvantages of Information Technology in Home Care

It is seldom the case that a system within an organization has only advantages and no disadvantages. Disadvantages related to information technology will be discussed from the point of view of both the care deliverers and the clients. Acceptance of technology in home care has, for some, been difficult. Some home care agencies have anticipated that their older nurses may be reluctant to learn the computer technology that is necessary to implement POC documentation. Some nurses have said they simply do not like being delegated to machines (Kinsella, 2003; Kobb et al., 2003).

Implementation of technology, especially POC documentation, is a process that takes several months depending on nurses' previous experience and comfort levels with computers. With proficiency, nurses have acknowledged that although client admissions require more time to complete than before POC, the admission note is more descriptive and access to the notes of other team members and better communication with clients outweigh the time issue (Struk, 2002a; Thoman et al., 2001).

Many nurses have learned that their clients do not feel that time has been taken away from them or feel otherwise deprived by their nurse's use of a laptop. Clients have said that they are comfortable with continuing conversation while their nurse is entering data, and others have agreed that computer technology in home care is becoming a necessity (Stricklin, Phelphs, & McVey, 2001).

Since the enactment of the Balanced Budget Act of 1997, home care agencies have had to find ways to increase the efficiency of their operations while maintaining quality client care. Telemonitoring may be one answer. Fewer in-person visits are required to monitor a client's status, thus reducing providers' time and mileage. A reduction in lengths of stay because of tele-monitoring may make a home care agency attractive to managed care organizations, thereby increasing partnerships (Averwater & Burchfield, 2005). However, financing a telemonitoring program can be costly for a home health agency. Help with funding may be available from government grants or from charitable organizations such as the United Way or private organizations such as the American Heart Association (Averwater & Burchfield, 2005).

Many issues related to computer technology in home care can be successfully overcome with development of a step-by-step curriculum, implementation of ongoing training programs, and an ongoing effort to keep personnel involved with the system. Ultimately success comes from nurses having more communication with their clients (Hockenjos & Wharton, 2001; Struk, 2002a; Thoman et al., 2001).

Looking to the Future

Advancements in telecommunications have changed and continue to change the delivery of health care. Governmental providers as well as private providers are predicting and planning for future telecommunication innovations.

Governmental Influences

Then-Secretary of the U. S. Department of Health and Human Services (USDHHS), Tommy Thompson, in July 2004, issued a news release announcing the formation of a 10-year plan to build a new health information infrastructure, and appointed Dr. David Brailer as the National Coordinator for Health Information Technology. The system, which is proposed to link health records electronically nationwide, motivated Secretary Thompson to state that "electronic health information will provide a quantum leap in client power, doctor power, and effective health care" (USDHHS, 2004, p. 1). In the Fall of 2005, contracts were awarded to accelerate the process of achieving the 10-year goal of interoperable electronic health records (USHHS, 2005).

Medicare payment for telehealth services is now available to physicians, hospitals, rural health clinics, and federally qualified health centers for distant site services to Medicare beneficiaries (USHHS, 2003). The future may see the addition of home care agencies to the current list of originating authorized sites.

Nongovernmental Influences

Home care providers have made predictions related to health care informatics. These predictions, based on home care trends, include a future where small palmtop commuters powerful as desktops, will replace laptops for point-of-care documentation. The palmtops will allow home care nurses instant access to all health information related to their clients. The size of diagnostic equipment is also expected to decrease, allowing home care nurses the ability to test clients at distant sites for specific conditions (Tweed, 2003).

In the following quote, the American Nurses Association succinctly predicts the future of nursing informatics:

> The speed of information transfer and the increasing availability of communications technologies will impact nurses and informatics nurse specialists in the future, making nursing practice and nursing informatics in particular, more international in practice with worldwide standards, competencies and curricula. (2001, p. 31.)

Summary

Nursing informatics and technology have entered the mainstream of delivery of health care to home care clients. Once delegated to acute care settings, information technology has become the system of choice for the collection, communication, and storage of client health data.

This chapter has discussed the history of nursing informatics and the types of information technology currently in use in home care settings. Particular attention has been given to point-of-care documentation. Attitudes and feelings of clients and providers towards information technology have been explored, and a look was given to the future of information technology in home care.

References

American Nurses Association. (2001). *Scope and practice of nursing informatics practice.* Washington, DC: American Nurses Publishing.

Averwater, N. W., & Burchfield, D. C. (2005). No place like home: Telemonitoring can improve home care. *Healthcare Financial Management, 59*(4), 46-48, 50-52.

Chetney, R. (2003a). Home care technology and telehealth—the future is here! *Home Healthcare Nurse, 21*(10), 645-646.

Chetney, R. (2003b). The cardiac connection program. *Home Healthcare Nurse, 21*(10), 680-686.

Dimmick, S. L., Burgiss, S. G., Robbins, S., Black, D., Jarnagin, B., & Anders, M. (2004). Outcomes of an integrated telehealth network demonstration project. *Telemedicine Journal and e-health, 9*(1), 13-23.

Hill, W., Weinert, C., & Cudney, S. (2006). Influence of a computer intervention on the psychological status of chronically ill rural women. *Nursing Research, 55*(1), 34-42.

Hockenjos, G. J., & Wharton, A. (2001). Point-of-care training: Strategies for success. *Home Healthcare Nurse, 19*(12), 766-773.

Jerant, A. F., Azari, R., & Nesbitt, T. S. (2001). Reducing the cost of frequent hospital admissions for congestive heart failure: A randomized trial of home telecare intervention. *Medical Care: A Journal of the American Public Health Association, 39*(11), 1234-1245.

Joch, A. (2003, Sept.). Wired for home care. *Homecare Informatics.* Retrieved August 4, 2004, from http://www.healthcare-informatics.com

Joint Commission on the Accreditation of Healthcare Organizations (JCAHO). (2005). Home care national patient safety goals. Retrieved October 7, 2005, from http://www.jcaho.org/accredited+organizations/patient+safety/06_npsg/06_npsg_ome.htm

Kinsella, A. (2003). Telehealth opportunities for home care clients. *Home Healthcare Nurse, 21*(10), 661–665.

Kobb, R., Hilsen, P., & Ryan, P. (2003). Assessing technology needs for the elderly. *Home Healthcare Nurse, 21*(10), 666–673.

Lewis, C. (2001). Emerging trends in medical device technology: Home is where the heart monitor is. *FDA Consumer Magazine, 35*(3). Retrieved August 4, 2005, from
http://www.fda.gov/fdac/fdacindex.html

Long, C. O., Greenberg, E. A., Ismeurt, R. L., & Smith, G. (2000). Computer and internet use by home care and hospice agencies. *Home Healthcare Nurse, 18*(10), 666–672.

Lupoli, J., & Rizzo, V. M. (2003). The impact of technology on the older nurse. *Home Healthcare Nurse, 21*(10), 691–692.

Mignor, D. L. (2000). Effectiveness of use of home health nurses to decrease burden & depression of elderly caregivers. *Journal of Psychosocial Nursing and Mental Health Services, 38*(7), 34–41.

National Alliance for Caregiving and AARP. (2004). *Caregiving in the U.S.* Retrieved August 12, 2004, from
http://www.caregiving.org/04finalreport.pdf

Russo, H. (2001). Window of opportunity for home care nurses. *Online Journal of Issues in Nursing, 6*(3), Manuscript 4. Available at
http://www.nursingworld.org/ojin/topic16/tpc14_4.htm

Saba, V. K. (2001). Nursing informatics: Yesterday, today and tomorrow. *International Nursing Review, 48*(3), 177–188.

Smith-Stoner, M. (2003). 10 uses for personal digital assistants in home care. *Home Healthcare Nurse, 21*(12), 797–800.

Stazesky, R. (2003). Lean, mean, data machine. *Health Management Technology, 24*(9), 28–29.

Stricklin, M. L. V., Niles, S. A., Struk, C., & Jones, S. (2000). What nurses and managers expect from point-of-care technology. *Home Healthcare Nurse, 18*(8), 515–523.

Stricklin, M. L. V., Phelphs, K. L., & McVey, R. J. (2001). Home care nurses' responses to point-of-care technology. *Home Healthcare Nurse, 19*(12), 774–778.

Struk, C. (2002a). The end user of home care computer technology: The clinician. *Home Healthcare Nurse, 20*(7), 466–469.

Struk, C. (2002b). Frequently asked questions about computer technology for clinicians. *Home Healthcare Nurse, 20*(12), 811–813.

Struk, C. (2001). Critical steps for integrating information technology in home care: One agency's experience. *Home Healthcare Nurse, 19*(12), 758–765.

Thoman, J., Struk, C., Spero, M. O., & Stricklin, M. L. (2001). Reflections from a point-of-care pilot nurse group experience. *Home Healthcare Nurse, 19*(12), 779–784.

Tweed, S. C. (2003). 7 performance-accelerating technologies that will shape the future of home care. *Home Healthcare Nurse, 21*(10), 647–650.

U.S. Department of Health & Human Services. (2005). HHS awards contracts to advance nationwide interoperable health information technology. Retrieved October 24, 2006, from
http://www.hhs.gov/news

U.S. Department of Health & Human Services. (2004). *Thompson launches "decade of health information technology."* Retrieved August 3, 2004, from
http://www.hhs.gov/news

U.S. Department of Health & Human Services. (2003). *Medicare payment for telehealth services* (Medicare Carriers Manual Part 3-Claims Process #1798). Rockwell, MD: Author. Retrieved July 31, 2004, from
http://www.cms.hhs.gov/manuals/pm_trans/R1798B.3.pdf

Glossary

Access Device The mechanism by which fluids are infused through the venous system into the body.

Advance Directives Instructions made by individuals expressing their wishes concerning their medical care prior to actually needing the care.

Antecedent Phase The preplanning phrase of a home visit that refers to the assessment aimed at assuring home care workers will be safe when entering a home. This phrase includes gathering as much information as possible including an assessment of the environment (both home and community) and the client's personal knowledge, skills, and competencies.

Bioethics Ethical issues that are specific to the field of health care.

Certification The process by which a physician assures that the client does have a medical condition that requires skilled care. The form sent to the physician to establish this need is referred to as HCFA-485.

Community-Acquired Methicillin-Resistant *Staphylococcus Aureus* A strain of *Staphylococcus aureus,* resistant to special beta-lactam drugs, that has been largely confined to hospitals and long-term facilities but is now emerging in the community.

Contact Precautions Precautions that are used to interrupt person-to-person transmission of organisms that are transmitted by direct or indirect contact with the skin. Contact precautions are built on the concept of standard precautions and are the most commonly used transmission precautions in home care.

Direct Observation Therapy A program used with known TB clients to ensure client compliance with TB medication regimes.

Distant Site The site where the health care provider is located to provide a health care service via a telecommunication system.

Environmental Props Factors in the environment that can be used to protect home care workers from harm.

Ethics The branch of philosophy that is involved with proposing, analyzing, and describing how humans ought to be and act.

Geographics The environmental context of the location in which a home visit occurs.

Governing Body (of a Home Care Agency) The designated persons who have the ultimate legal authority and responsibility for the overall operation of the agency.

Hand Hygiene The process of cleaning a health care worker's hands with soap and water or alcohol gel at prescribed times.

Home Health Agency A public or private agency or organization that is primarily engaged in providing skilled nursing services and other therapeutic services such as physical therapy, speech-language therapy, or occupational therapy; has policies established by a professional group including at least one physician and one registered nurse; is licensed in accordance with state or local law; and meets other conditions found by the Secretary of Health and Human Services to be necessary for health and safety.

Home care That component of a continuum of comprehensive health care in which health care services are provided to individuals and families in their place of residence, usually their home, for the purpose of maximizing their level of independence; promoting, maintaining, and restoring health; or facilitating a comfortable death.

Home care Nurse Educator A registered nurse, employed by a home care agency, who in the course of providing skilled nursing care to clients is teaching the client, caregiver, and family that which they need to know to provide optimal care.

Human Resources The individuals who are employed by an organization.

Informatics Computer processing of data and information.

Infusion Therapy The administration of fluids or medications into the body through the intravenous, subcutaneous, or epidural routes.

The Joint Commission (JC), formerly the Joint Commission on Accreditation of Health care Organizations (JCAHO) The national accreditors for health care.

Leadership Team (of a Home care Agency) The group of people who are responsible for providing the overall direction for the agency. The team's responsibilities include planning, budgeting, performance improvement, and customer relations.

Literacy The ability to read, write, and speak English proficiently; to compute and solve problems; and to use technology in order to become a life-long learner and be effective in the family, the workplace, and the community.

Malpractice Professional misconduct, unreasonable lack of skill, or fidelity in professional or judicial duties.

Medicaid A state medical assistance program, established at the same time as Medicare, that provides for some home care services. Medicaid is primarily used by the poor or uninsured.

Medicare Health care legislation passed in 1965 as part of President Lyndon Johnson's "Great Society" initiative. The legislation includes home care benefits, primarily skilled nursing and therapy of a curative or restorative nature.

Methicillin-resistant *Staphylococcus Aureus* (MRSA) A strain of *Staphylococcus aureus* that is resistant to special beta-lactam drugs that are used to treat these organisms.

Morality How people actually behave.

Negligence The failure to exercise the degree of care that a person of ordinary prudence would exercise under the same circumstances. Negligence includes not doing something that should have been done as well as doing something that should not have been done.

Nurse Practice Acts A set of statements that defines the practice of nursing, gives guidance for the scope of practice, and sets standards for the nursing profession.

Nursing Ethics The process in nursing that proposes, analyzes, and describes ways that nurses ought to be and act regarding bioethical issues and nurses' everyday work.

Nursing Informatics The process in nursing that processes information and transforms data from input data to output information via computer technology and computer systems.

Nursing Practice The performance by nurses of skills and services for the purpose of assisting people in the pursuit of wellness, or through illness and/or death.

Outcome The cumulative effect at a defined point in time of performing one or more processes in the care of a client.

Outcomes and Assessment Information Set (OASIS) A group of uniform data sets designed to evaluate the consistency and quality of care provided and to quality the outcomes of home care.

Per Visit Staff Organizational employees or contract employees who are paid by client visit.

Performance Improvement The study and adaptation of functions and processes to increase the probability of achieving desired outcomes.

Personal Protective Equipment Equipment (gowns, gloves, and masks) worn by health care workers that act as barriers to prevent and control infection.

Plan of Care A client plan that consists of the physician's orders, the comprehensive assessment, the available agency reimbursement, the treatment needed, and the discipline necessary to deliver the treatment.

Point-of-care The immediate documentation of client care, usually via a laptop, that results in the documentation being recorded at the time of the client's care thus at the point-of-care.

Preceptor A professional employed in a practice setting who is assigned to work along side of a student or a new employee for the purpose of teaching/learning.

Pulmonary Tuberculosis An infectious disease caused by *Mycobacterium tuberculosis* that is spread through airborne particles.

Quality The degree to which health services for individuals and populations increase the likelihood that desired health outcomes are consistent with current professional knowledge.

Recognized Hazards Any act, incident, or serious situation that poses a threat to people physically, emotionally, socially, economically, or spiritually.

Referral The physician's order for a client assessment or evaluation for the need of skilled home care.

Regular Staff Organizational employees who are either salaried or paid by the hour.

Risk Adjustment The process of compensation or controlling for the potential influence of risk factors or case mix variables that can affect outcomes.

Safety Freedom from danger.

Scope of Practice The permissible boundaries of practice for the health professional as defined by rules and regulations.

Scope of Service The types of services a home care agency provides.

Skilled Care Care that only a registered nurse, registered physical therapist, or registered language therapist can provide.

Standard Precautions Precautions that direct the health care worker to treat all human blood and body fluids as if they are infected with pathogens. Standard precautions were previously known as universal precautions.

Standards of Practice The levels or degrees of quality considered adequate by a given profession. Standards of practice are the skills and learning commonly possessed by members of a profession.

Teaching/learning The process of assessing what is needed to know (by the learner), evaluating the learner's readiness to know, setting learning goals, and providing a mechanism to learn (by the teacher) that ultimately changes behavior.

Telehealth Remote care that is delivered or monitored between a health care provider and a client outside of a clinical health facility, usually the home.

Total Parental Nutrition (TPN) The infusion of a solution directly into a vein to meet the client's daily nutritional requirements.

Index

Note: Page numbers followed by "f" indicate figures, those followed by "t" indicate tables, and those followed by "b" indicate boxes.